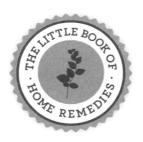

ACHES
— *and* —
AILMENTS

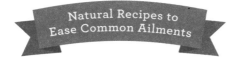

Natural Recipes to
Ease Common Ailments

Linda B. White, M.D.
Barbara H. Seeber & Barbara Brownell Grogan

© 2015 Fair Winds Press
Text © 2014 Linda B. White, M.D., Barbara Brownell Grogan, and Barbara H. Seeber

First published in the USA in 2015 by
Fair Winds Press, a member of
Quarto Publishing Group USA Inc.
100 Cummings Center
Suite 406-L
Beverly, MA 01915-6101
www.fairwindspress.com
Visit www.bodymindbeautyhealth.com. It's your personal guide to a happy, healthy, and extraordinary life!

19 18 17 16 15   2 3 4 5

ISBN: 978-1-59233-670-8

Content for this book was previously published in the book 500 *Time-Tested Home Remedies and the Science Behind Them* by Linda B. White, M.D., Barbara Brownell Grogan, and Barbara H. Seeber (Fair Winds Press, 2014).

Cover design by Leigh Ring // RingArtDesign.com
Book design by Leigh Ring // RingArtDesign.com

The information in this book is for educational purposes only. It is not intended to replace the advice of a physician or medical practitioner. Please see your health care provider before beginning any new health program. The authors and publisher are not responsible for readers' misuse of these recipes and, as a result, any unintended effects.

Printed and bound in the USA

Contents

Introduction

In today's high-powered, health-conscious world, we're all smarter, more informed about our bodies, and preoccupied with ways to live long, healthy lives. We've accomplished half of that goal: living longer. But we're missing the "living healthier" part of the equation.

On December 15, 2012, the British medical journal *The Lancet* published data from the Global Burden of Disease Study 2010. Here are the key findings, starting with the good news: Around the world, longevity has increased. We're less likely to succumb prematurely to malaria and measles, but more likely to drop dead later in life from heart attack or stroke. The bad news is, we're more likely to spend our last years disabled by diseases—most of which are preventable.

Chronic illness has long dogged Americans. Now it's spreading to other countries. Where have we gone wrong? We have health-related facts and figures at our fingertips. We have expensive diagnostic tests, highly trained doctors, and cutting-edge treatments. The shelves in supermarkets groan under the weight of boxes, cans, and bags. Modern conveniences have reduced our need for physical labor. Computers give us up-to-date medical bulletins.

Despite these advances, and to some extent because of them, we've become fat, flabby, and frequently ill. We're too often hurried, harried, sleep-deprived, and socially disconnected. We eat in our cars, at our desks, in front of televisions—everywhere but at the dining room table in the company of others. We sit too much and move too little.

It turns out that health springs largely from old-fashioned behaviors—eating wholesome food, enjoying friends, relaxing, getting enough sleep, moving our bodies, and using natural remedies to heal.

The goal of this book is to help you get back to the basic lifestyle measures that point you toward a healthy, vibrant future.

We provide lots of practical information on preventing and managing ailments. You'll find time-tested recipes and lifestyle tips—all designed to give you sometimes quick, always natural, ways to soothe, calm, and heal.

We hope you enjoy this book. May it enlighten you, guiding you along natural and simple paths to your healthy future.

Asthma

Each day, nine Americans die during an asthma attack. Unfortunately, an increasing number of Americans have asthma. The current count is about 25 million people. Asthma has become the most common chronic disease in childhood. Theories about the rise in asthma include changes in dietary habits, environmental pollutants, indoor lifestyles, and an increase in obesity.

This inflammatory condition usually begins in childhood. African-American and Puerto Rican children are at particularly high risk. Symptoms include a cough that's typically worse at night and in the early morning, chest tightness, wheezing, shortness of breath, and increased respiratory rate. The airways become inflamed, swollen, constricted, and congested with excess mucus. It's like trying to breathe through a straw.

A combination of genetic predisposition and environmental factors causes asthma. Part of the treatment involves identifying and avoiding (or preparing for) triggers.

Medications don't cure asthma; rather, they help keep the condition under control. The drug regimen depends upon whether the symptoms are intermittent or persistent. Inhaled bronchodilators open the airway to nip an attack in the bud. For persistent asthma, inhaled anti-inflammatory medications are taken daily. It's important to follow the treatment plan. That said, a number of foods and exercises can gently and safely support lung health.

Natural asthma remedies include acupuncture, chiropractic treatments, massage therapy, biofeedback, homeopathy, dietary improvements, and dietary supplements, such as herbs, vitamins, and minerals. Research supporting these therapies is preliminary at best. Science has yet to discover a cure for asthma—natural or otherwise. Kids sometimes grow out of it— that is, stop being symptomatic as their lungs grow bigger.

Such remedies as deep abdominal breathing, progressive muscle relaxation, guided imagery, biofeedback, and regular massage can help relieve emotional stress, which can aggravate asthma. Dietary changes are important for avoiding known food triggers and maximizing intake of natural antioxidants.

Omega-Packed Salmon Fillets

Don't overdo the baking time, or your fish will be dry and unappealing. If you keep it pink in the center and cook it until it just flakes at the touch of a fork, this omega-3 powerhouse is divine.

2 salmon fillets (6 to 8 ounces, or 170 to 225 g each)

2 teaspoons (10 ml) olive oil

1 to 2 tablespoons (14 g) bread crumbs ½ teaspoon dried tarragon

1 tablespoon (15 g) Dijon mustard Pinch of paprika

Lemon slices, for garnish

PREPARATION AND USE:

Preheat the oven to 450°F (230°C, or gas mark 8). Rinse the salmon fillets and pat them dry. Lightly grease a glass baking dish with the olive oil. Place the fish skin side down in the dish. Mix the tarragon into the mustard and spread over the fish. Sprinkle each fillet with the bread crumbs and paprika. Bake for 10 to 15 minutes until just past pink in the center. Top with the lemon slices and serve.

YIELD: 2 servings

❓ **How it works:** The omega-3 fatty acids in high-oil fish, such as salmon, sardines, tuna, and mackerel, are anti-inflammatory. Studies suggest that diets higher in the omega-3 fatty acids found in fish oil may improve asthma.

Antioxidant-Rich Waldorf Salad

6 tablespoons (75 g) plain Greek yogurt

2 tablespoons (28 ml) fresh lemon juice

1/8 teaspoon each sea salt and freshly ground black pepper

1 cup (100 g) chopped celery

1 cup (150 g) sliced seedless red grapes

2 large red sweet apples, peeled, cored, and chopped

1 cup (100 g) walnuts Pinch of paprika

Celery leaves, for garnish

PREPARATION AND USE:

In a large bowl, whip the yogurt and lemon juice together. Stir in the salt and pepper. In a separate bowl, mix the celery, grapes, apple, and walnuts. Pour the yogurt mixture over the fruit mixture until covered. Stir to combine. Add a pinch of paprika to each serving. Garnish with the celery leaves.

YIELD: 4 servings

❓ **How it works:** Apples, grapes, and celery leaves are high in flavonoids (water-soluble plant pigments that benefit health) and vitamin C. Both are antioxidant. People with chronic lung conditions, such as asthma, often have low levels of antioxidants, perhaps because this inflammatory condition depletes them. One study found that vitamin C supplementation helped protect against exercise-induced asthma. Others studies have shown that more fresh fruit in the diet improves asthma. Also, the beneficial bacteria in yogurt promote gut health. Research increasingly suggests that abnormal resident "flora," or bacteria, predispose people to asthma and other allergic conditions. Preliminary research suggests that some probiotic supplements improve airway responses.

Carotene Booster

Autumn is the perfect time of year to enjoy those colorful, carotene-rich pumpkins, which are members of the squash family.

1 pumpkin (3 pounds, or 1.36 kg) washed, cut in half, and seeded

⅓ cup (80 ml) olive oil

2 tablespoons (28 ml) balsamic vinegar 1 teaspoon (2 g) ground cinnamon

1 teaspoon (7 g) honey

1 tablespoon (14 g) unsalted butter

PREPARATION AND USE:
Preheat the oven to 425°F (220°C, or gas mark 7). Cut the pumpkin into ten wedges. Put the wedges on a baking sheet. Mix the olive oil and vinegar together, pour over the pumpkin, and toss until the pumpkin is covered. Spread the wedges in a single layer across the sheet. Sprinkle each wedge with cinnamon. Roast for about 40 minutes. Remove from the oven and top the inside of each wedge with a tiny pat of butter. Enjoy the pumpkin by scooping it out of the skin.

YIELD: 4-6 servings

❓ How it works: Pumpkins, yellow squash, carrots, bell peppers, and other orange-hued vegetables and fruits get their pigment from carotenoids, powerful antioxidants that reduce inflammation, support the immune system, and maintain respiratory linings. One study found that a supplement containing a mixture of carotenes helped to prevent exercise-induced asthma.

Iced Coffee Pick-Me-Up

We love this drink for a late morning boost; try to enjoy it before noon, especially if caffeine keeps you awake at night.

2 cups (475 ml) water

$\frac{1}{4}$ cup (55 g) ground dark roast coffee

$\frac{1}{4}$ cup (78 g) sweetened condensed milk,

divided 8 ice cubes

PREPARATION AND USE:

Brew the coffee. Pour half of the condensed milk into each of two mugs. Divide the hot coffee between the mugs. Stir until the milk is dissolved. Fill two tall glasses with four ice cubes each. Gradually pour each portion of hot coffee over the ice and stir to chill (for a thinner, cooler drink, add more cubes). Enjoy!

YIELD: 2 servings

Recipe Variation: On chilly days, try this coffee hot—just leave out the ice cubes and add a pinch of ground cinnamon.

❓ **How it works:** Several studies have shown that caffeine modestly improves lung function for up to 4 hours in people with asthma. Avoid late afternoon or evening intake, which could interfere with a good night's sleep. Caffeine is related to theophylline, an asthma medication that helps open airways, reducing breathlessness.

Eucalyptus Chest Rub

The smell alone of this soothing rub brings respiratory relief.

1 tablespoon (15 ml) unscented lotion, olive oil, or (15 g) petroleum jelly

2 drops eucalyptus essential oil

PREPARATION AND USE:

Blend the lotion and essential oil in a small, clean jar. Rub the mixture onto your chest: Start with a small amount to see how you respond to eucalyptus. Inhale deeply as you work. You're drawing some of those aromatic, medicinal oils into your lungs. Wash your hands thoroughly before touching your eyes, nose, or other sensitive mucous membranes. If you have any remaining rub, store it in the jar and cap tightly.

YIELD: 1 rub

❓ **How it works:** Eucalyptus has anti-inflammatory, expectorant effects. It may also help open the airways by relaxing the encircling muscles. One study found that a special preparation taken internally eased asthma symptoms and reduced the need for medications. However, it is not safe to take eucalyptus essential oil by mouth. Plant essential oils are highly concentrated. Many are toxic when taken internally.

Beneficial Tuna with Brazil Nuts

Once you've enjoyed this dish hot from the oven, keep up your omega-3s by putting the leftovers in tuna salad sandwiches (mix with plain yogurt and a little lemon instead of mayonnaise).

4 tuna medallions (4 ounces, or 115 g each) 2 teaspoons (10 ml) olive oil

$1/4$ teaspoon sea salt

Freshly ground black pepper, to taste

$1/4$ cup (33 g) crushed Brazil nuts Lemon wedges, for garnish

PREPARATION AND USE:

Preheat the oven to 425°F (220°C, or gas mark 7). Rinse the tuna medallions and pat dry. Brush each side with olive oil and sprinkle with salt and pepper. Roll the medallions in the crushed nuts. Coat a glass baking dish with vegetable oil spray. Bake the tuna for 15 to 20 minutes until the center is just past pink.

YIELD: 4 servings

❓ **How it works:** Brazil nuts and seafood are excellent sources of selenium, an antioxidant that works against inflammation. At least two studies have shown that people who consumed selenium in their diet were less likely to have asthma than were those who did not. Tuna is a good source of omega-3 fatty acids, which help reduce inflammation in airways. One survey showed that families that ate oily fish high in omega-3s, such as tuna, sardines, and salmon, had a nearly three times' lower percentage of children with asthma than families that did not.

Beneficial Turmeric Toddy

Enjoy this soothing beverage throughout the day, especially before bed.

1 cup (235 ml) milk

1 teaspoon (2 g) ground turmeric

PREPARATION AND USE:

Heat the milk to your desired warmth, but do not boil it. Stir in the turmeric. Drink this mixture up to three times daily.

YIELD: 1 serving

❓ **How it works:** This Indian spice is a potent anti-inflammatory agent. Preliminary research suggests that concentrated extracts of turmeric and other anti-inflammatory herbs can improve some aspects of asthma. The fat in milk can improve intestinal absorption of curcumin, the active ingredient in turmeric.

WHEN SIMPLE DOESN'T WORK

Preliminary research suggests that standardized, concentrated extracts of some herbs may hold modest benefits for people with asthma. They include ginkgo, coleus, long pepper, curcumin (an active ingredient in turmeric), and pycnogenol (from French maritime pine). Herbalists often recommend horehound and mullein as general lung tonics. However, check with your health provider before taking any herbs or other dietary supplements.

Aussie Steam

Eucalyptus trees are native to Australia and have long been used to
manage coughs and asthma.

1 quart (946 ml) water

1 to 2 drops eucalyptus essential oil, or $\frac{1}{4}$ cup
(6 g) crushed, dried eucalyptus leaves

PREPARATION AND USE:

Boil the water. Turn off the heat. If using eucalyptus essential oil, remove
the pot from the burner. First try inhaling the steam. If steam alone doesn't
trigger asthmatic coughing, add 1 drop of eucalyptus oil. Lean in gradually.
If the eucalyptus vapors don't trigger coughing, you can add the second
drop of essential oil. Cover your head with a clean towel to entrap the steam.
Breathe through your mouth slowly and deeply for 1 to 2 minutes. If using
dried eucalyptus leaves, add them to the pot, cover, and steep for 10 to 15
minutes. Remove the lid. If you no longer have steam, heat the liquid again—
just to the boiling point—and remove from the burner. Lean over the steam
and cover your head with a clean towel. Breathe slowly and deeply. If the
steam triggers coughing or seems to worsen your asthma in any way, stop.

YIELD: 1 application

❓ How it works: Brazil nuts and seafood are excellent sources of
selenium, an antioxidant that works against inflammation. At least two
studies have shown that people who consumed selenium in their diet were
less likely to have asthma than were those who did not. Tuna is a good
source of omega-3 fatty acids, which help reduce inflammation in airways.
One survey showed that families that ate oily fish high in omega-3s, such
as tuna, sardines, and salmon, had a nearly three times' lower percentage
of children with asthma than families that did not.

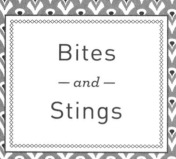

Bites
—and—
Stings

All manner of animals can bite. In terms of mammalian bites, the most likely offenders are cats, dogs, other humans, and rabid creatures, such as foxes, raccoons, bobcats, skunks, and bats. By law, owners should vaccinate dogs, cats, and pet ferrets, though not everyone complies.

If you're bitten, someone—not you—should catch the animal so it can be tested for rabies. Call the police or state health department for assistance. The last thing you need is to be further injured and emotionally traumatized.

If the bite is deep or extensive, call 911. Otherwise, your first step is to wash the wound with soap and copious amounts of running water. If you keep povidone-iodine (an antiseptic chemical complex that contains iodine and is stocked in most drugstores) on hand, apply that, too (check the label to see whether it first should be diluted). Stanch bleeding by applying pressure and then a sterile bandage.

Seek medical attention for all bites that break the skin, especially human bites, which are most likely to become severely infected, and bites to the hands and face. In addition to having the wound properly treated, you may need a tetanus booster. If the animal has rabies (or couldn't be caught and is presumed to have rabies), you may also need a rabies immune globulin injection and a four-part rabies vaccine. The rabies immune globulin is injected into the wound and surrounding tissue. In case you've heard tell of the vaccine being injected into the belly, rest assured that the vaccine is injected into the muscle in the upper arm or in the case of small children, the thigh.

RECIPES TO TREAT BITES AND STINGS

Unstick the Tick

Make a thorough body search after a summer walk in the woods—and have the items below handy. If bitten, follow the instructions.

Soap and water

Antibiotic ointment

PREPARATION AND USE:

With tweezers, carefully grasp the tick as close to your skin as possible. Gently pull until the tick comes free (do not twist or jerk, as the head may break off and remain embedded). Wash thoroughly, pat dry, and apply the antibiotic ointment. Save the tick in a resealable plastic bag and place in the freezer, in case medical staff later request it for identification. If mouthparts remain behind, see your doctor. Wash your hands well and clean the tweezers to disinfect from the tick.

YIELD: 1 application

❓ **How it works:** Careful removal of the tick, immediate cleansing, and application of antibiotic ointment will prevent topical infection. Prompt removal of the tick can reduce the risk of transmission of such diseases as Lyme disease.

Quick Clean: Human, Dog, or Cat Bites

When you're bitten, cleaning is just part of the care; follow all the important steps below.

Warm water

Soap

Antibacterial ointment

PREPARATION AND USE:

With a clean cloth, apply direct pressure to stop the bleeding. Once the bleeding slows, rinse the wound with running water (by holding the area under the tap). Then dip a second clean cloth into the warm water, rub with soap, and clean the wound thoroughly. Rinse again. Pat dry. Apply an antibacterial ointment and cover the wound with a sterile bandage. Clean the wound and change the bandage every day—sooner if it gets dirty, wet, or bloody.

Next, call your doctor's office to find out whether your injury warrants prompt medical treatment. Cat bites count as puncture wounds, which means they're at higher risk for becoming infected. You also want to check that your tetanus shot is up to date. If any wound is deep (or 10 to 15 minutes of steady pressure doesn't stop the bleeding), proceed to the emergency room. In the event of severe injury, call 911.

YIELD: 1 application

❓ **How it works:** Running water flushes out microbes.Washing with soap and water and applying an antibacterial ointment further reduce the risk of subsequent infection.

Bee Stinger Removal

Don't let that venom sink in!

Ice cube

Warm water

Soap

PREPARATION AND USE:

As quickly as possible, remove the stinger by gently scraping it off with your fingernail, a credit card, or another stiff object. Grasp an ice cube and rub it briskly over the stung area for a full minute. Wash with warm water and soap. If you're stung on the arm, remove rings and bracelets before swelling occurs.

YIELD: 1 application

❓ How it works: A bee usually leaves behind a sac of venom and a stinger. Removing it immediately stops more venom from entering. Cleansing the site wards off infection. Keep the area clean during the healing process, which may take up to five days.

❗ Warning: Do not pinch or pull the stinger; this can inject more venom.

Bee-lieve the Relief

College student Candice McCay keeps bees in Denver. She and her husband find this recipe helpful in relieving pain and swelling.

Water

5 drops lavender essential oil

PREPARATION AND USE:

Wet a washcloth with water and wring out the excess moisture. Dot on the lavender essential oil. Seal the washcloth in a resealable freezer bag and store in the freezer at the beginning of bee season. It will be good for the summer months. Replace it with a fresh one when it's used. If you're stung, remove the cloth from the bag and apply it directly to the area.

YIELD: 1 application

❓ **How it works:** Ice reduces swelling and relieves pain. Lavender is anti-inflammatory, analgesic, and calming.

De-Itcher

This remedy is a quick and easy fix for bee and fire ant stings.

1 teaspoon (4.6 g) baking soda
3 drops lavender essential oil
Water

PREPARATION AND USE:

Put the baking soda in your palm. Add the lavender essential oil and enough water to form a paste. Plaster the paste over the sting site, covering the swelling. After 30 minutes, rinse off the paste. Reapply as needed.

YIELD: 1 application

❓ **How it works:** Bee and fire ant stings are acidic, though the venom contains other chemicals at well. The baking soda paste may help neutralize the acidic venom. As noted above, lavender decreases inflammation, pain, and anxiety.

Honey Fix for Stings or Bites

This remedy is appropriate for any bite or sting that doesn't require emergency medical attention.

1 teaspoon (7 g) honey

PREPARATION AND USE:

Apply the honey to the bite site so it is fully covered. Leave in place for 30 minutes and then rinse. Reapply as needed.

YIELD: 1 application

❷ How it works: Honey is an ancient wound healer that has recently garnered scientific support for its antibacterial and anti-inflammatory effects. Studies show it improves the healing of cuts, scrapes, burns, and other wounds.

Bruises

Life is full of bumps and bruises. When we learn to crawl, walk, ride a bike, stand on our hands, or skate—anytime we push the envelope of our physical capabilities, we risk falling. It's how we learn and gain new skills. Of course, we also bruise ourselves in embarrassing ways. When hurried, harried, and distracted, your own house can become a minefield. Bruises can result from surgical procedures and accidental injuries—slips on icy walks, car crashes, and so forth.

No matter how you sustain one, a bruise (also called a contusion) represents soft tissue trauma. Skin turns plum-colored because burst blood vessels have spilled red blood cells into the surrounding tissue. Later, breakdown products from those cells create green and yellow hues. Extra fluid in the tissues causes swelling. And, unfortunately, there's some degree of tenderness. Deeper bruising of muscle and the lining of bones may be particularly painful.

If you bump your head, you can end up with an "egg." That bump indicates that a blood vessel tore under the scalp. You can also bruise your brain. Although both stem from physical trauma, brain contusions aren't the same as brain concussions. The former involves a localized bruising. Concussions affect the brain more globally and microscopically. For instance, if someone rear-ends your car, the forward and backward motion of your head causes your brain to bobble, striking the inside of the skull as it does.

RECIPES TO TREAT BRUISES

Cold Pack

6 ice cubes, crushed

PREPARATION AND USE:

Place the ice in a resealable plastic bag. Wrap in a clean cloth. Apply to the bruised area for 15 to 20 minutes. Repeat at least three times a day.

YIELD: 1 application

? How it works: Immediate application of an ice pack can help slow, or even prevent, swelling from a bruise.

LIFESTYLE TIP

Peas, please. Keep a pack of frozen peas in the fridge. It's a good alternative for the ice pack above. Apply for 10 to 15 minutes when a bruise starts to burgeon.

Elevation Salvation

This is for serious bruising. Minor bruises, from bumping into a chair or table, for example, don't cause much swelling.

3 pillows

Your bruised area

An ice pack (see Cold Pack, at left)

PREPARATION AND USE:

Sit or lie in a comfortable position. Pile up the pillows in a strategic place. Rest the bruised arm, leg, foot, or head against the pillows so that the area is above heart level. Apply the ice pack. Practice this as often as possible when injury first occurs.

YIELD: 1 application

❓ **How it works:** How it works: Keeping the bruised area above your heart level and applying ice will help minimize swelling.

Aloe Vera Gel

2 tablespoons (28 g) Aloe vera gel

1 tablespoon (6.8) ground turmeric

1 teaspoon ground ginger

2 drops peppermint essential oil

PREPARATION AND USE:

In a small bowl, blend all the ingredients to form a paste. Apply to the skin, covering the bruise. Cover the paste with gauze or a clean cloth. Rest for 15 to 30 minutes. Remove the gauze and paste.

YIELD: 1 application

❓ **How it works:** How it works: Turmeric and ginger are both anti-inflammatory and analgesic. Peppermint reduces pain. Aloe vera is anti-inflammatory and speeds wound healing. Because aloe is readily absorbed into the skin, it may help drag other chemical ingredients along with it.

❗ **Warning:** Take care not to get this mixture on your clothes, as it will stain. Also, avoid contact with your eyes. The turmeric will temporarily turn your skin yellow.

Kale and Blueberry Salad

1 bunch kale, thinly sliced, minus stems

1 cup (145 g) blueberries

¼ red onion, sliced

1 cup (110 g) finely chopped pecans or (120 g)walnuts

1 tablespoon (15 g) fresh lime juice

1 tablespoon (15 g) fresh lemon juice

¼ cup (30 g) blue cheese

PREPARATION AND USE:

Toss the kale, blueberries, onion, and nuts in a large bowl. Mix the lemon and lime juice and add to the salad, coating all the pieces. Let the salad sit for about 10 minutes as the kale wilts. Toss in the blue cheese and serve.

YIELD: 4 main course servings, OR 8 side dish servings

❓ **How it works:** Vitamin K is essential for blood clotting. Good sources include leafy greens, such as kale, spinach, collard, and turnip greens, as well as asparagus. Vitamin C and flavonoids are needed for the production of collagen, a protein that keeps skin and blood vessels strong. All fresh fruits and vegetables contain them and blueberries in particular are an excellent source.

Pineapple Press

Cut open a fresh pineapple. Because canned pineapple undergoes pasteurization, which involves heat, the beneficial enzyme bromelain is lost.

1 fresh pineapple

PREPARATION AND USE:

Slice a piece of pineapple and apply the flesh to the bruise. Hold in place for 15 minutes. Meantime, eat as much pineapple as you like.

YIELD: 1 application

❓ **How it works:** Pineapple contains the enzyme bromelain, which reduces inflammation. In one study, bromelain (taken internally as a supplement) reduced pain and swelling after blunt trauma.

❗ **Warning:** If pineapple irritates your skin, don't use it.

Note: Alternatively, apply fresh pineapple juice to a clean cloth or piece of gauze and apply to the area for 5 to 10 minutes.

Witch to the Rescue

Witch hazel

PREPARATION AND USE:
Soak a clean cloth in witch hazel and apply directly to the bruise. Hold for 15 to 20 minutes, allowing the elixir to soak into the skin.

YIELD: 4 main course servings, OR 8 side dish servings

? How it works: Witch hazel is an astringent, meaning it contracts tissue to reduce bleeding and swelling.

LIFESTYLE TIP

Don't smoke! Smoking decreases blood circulation and retards wound healing.

Burns

Most anyone who spends much time in the kitchen or out in the sun has experienced a burn. Causes of burns include ultraviolet light, hot liquids, fire, electricity, and chemicals. Although the skin is normally involved, hot liquids can burn the mouth and throat; inhalation of smoke and some chemicals can burn the lungs.

Burns come in three varieties:

First-degree burns affect the epidermis, the outermost layer of skin. They cause redness and pain, and, after a couple of days, peeling skin.

Second-degree burns extend into the dermis, the bottom layer of skin. In addition to redness, pain, and swelling, they raise blisters.

Third-degree burns, also called full-thickness burns, destroy the skin and damage underlying tissues. Because nerves are damaged, the area may be numb. Other signs include white or charred skin.

If a first- or second-degree burn occurs, swiftly remove the skin from the source of heat. Plunge the area into cool water for five minutes. If clothing can't be quickly removed (or is stuck to the skin), thrust it into the water, too. Afterward, wash the area with mild soap and water and cover with sterile gauze. Remove any constricting jewelry from the area. If arms or legs are involved, elevate to about the level of the heart.

Once the injury has occurred, it can take twenty-four to forty-eight hours for the burn to stop progressing. Redness, blisters, and peeling will steadily evolve.

Burn Response 101

Burn victim

PREPARATION AND USE:

Pull the victim away from the fire, boiling liquid, or steam. If the victim is on fire, push him or her to the ground and roll his or her body to smother the flames. Pull away smoking material or charred clothing from victim. If clothing sticks to the skin, cut or tear around it. Immediately remove any jewelry, tight clothing, and restrictive accessories, such as belts, to prevent swelling.

To treat a first-degree burn (which affects only the top layer of skin): Hold the skin under cool water until the pain is relieved or apply cool compresses. Cover with a sterile, nonstick bandage or clean cloth and do not apply ointment. Whereas cool water dispels heat, the old-fashioned treatment with butter (a simple type of ointment) can actually hold in heat. Once the wound has cooled, antibacterial ointment or healing herbal salve is fine.

To treat a second-degree burn (which affects the top two layers of skin): Immerse the burn area in cool water for 10 to 15 minutes or apply cool compresses. Do not apply ice or submerge in an ice bath, as prolonged exposure to cold temperatures will further damage tissue. Cover loosely with a sterile, nonstick bandage and do not apply ointment.

If the second-degree burn covers a large part of the body, also: Lay the person flat. Elevate his or her feet by about 12 inches (30 cm). Raise the burn area above the heart level. Drape the victim with a blanket or warm clothing. Call the doctor immediately.

To treat a third-degree burn (which damages all layers of skin and may extend even deeper):

Call 911. Cover the area with a sterile, nonstick bandage, a sheet for larger areas, or any clean material that will not leave cloth in the wound. Separate the victim's fingers and toes with sterile cloth. Do not apply water or ointments.

YIELD: Different for each circumstance

❓ **How it works:** Burns require immediate attention. Assess the situation and act as set out above. Never take a chance. See a doctor immediately for second-degree burns. Dial 911 when a fire or other life-threatening situation causes third-degree burns.

Aloe-ah Burns

1 tablespoon (15 g) Aloe vera gel
 (Look for a product that's at least 90 percent aloe.)
10 drops lavender essential oil

PREPARATION AND USE:
Blend the aloe gel and essential oil to make a paste. Apply the paste as needed to the burn.

YIELD: Several applications for a small burn

❓ **How it works:** Aloe vera gel inhibits pain-producing substances. It is anti-inflammatory, promotes circulation, and inhibits bacteria and fungi. Studies show that it speeds healing of burns and wounds, improves psoriasis, and enhances tissue survival after frostbite. Although not all studies have been positive, cumulative research does indicate that topical aloe gel benefits firstand second-degree burns. Lavender essential oil is anti-inflammatory, pain-relieving, antibacterial, and antifungal.

Sweet Soother

Honey (a fresh, uncontaminated jar)

PREPARATION AND USE:

Blend the aloe gel and essential oil to make a paste. Apply the paste as needed to the burn.

YIELD: 1 application

? How it works: Honey is an ancient wound healer. Scientific studies show it's antibacterial and speeds healing of burns on par with the more conventional burn dressings containing silver sulfadiazine.

Note: Manuka honey is especially effective if you are concerned about skin infection. (It is available at health food stores and is expensive.)

Alternatively, mix a teaspoon of honey with a teaspoon of Aloe vera gel and apply to the gauze. You'll get double the healing action.

Oat Balm

6 tablespoons (30 g) rolled oats

¾ cup (175 ml) water

PREPARATION AND USE:

Combine the oats and water in a microwave-safe bowl. Microwave on high for 2 minutes or until cooked. Let cool. Cover the burned area with the cooled oat mixture. Wrap in clean muslin or gauze and keep it in place for 30 minutes to an hour.

YIELD: 1 application

❓ **How it works:** Oatmeal is soothing to burned skin. The gooeyness comes from a polysaccharide (complex sugar) called beta-glucan. It helps protect and hold water in the skin. Other compounds called phenols have antioxidant and anti-inflammatory activity.

Note: Alternatively, in coffee mill or food processor, grind ½ cup (40 g) of rolled oats to a powder and add to a tepid bath. If you don't want to grind the oats, put them in a sock and tie the top to avoid clogging your drain. Swish the sock around for 5 minutes before you step into the bathtub.

Calendula Tincture

2 teaspoons (1 g) dried calendula flowers (also called pot marigold,
  available at a natural food store)

1 cup (235 ml) boiling water

PREPARATION AND USE:

Steep the calendula flowers in the boiling water for 10 minutes. Strain and
let cool. Apply to the burn with a clean cloth. Repeat as often as possible.

YIELD: 1 or more applications

? How it works: The calendula flower is antiseptic and helps heal
wounds. It is also anti-inflammatory and cooling, which soothes a burn.

Fact or Myth?

IF YOU'RE BURNED, APPLY ICE.

Myth. Prolonged contact with ice and ice water can further
injure tissues and also may lead to hypothermia (abnormally
low body temperature). If, on the other hand, you burn your
hand in the kitchen, dunking it for 1 to 5 minutes into a cup of
ice water is fine.

Green Tea Cocktail

Burned skin loses its barrier function, allowing water to escape. Be sure to drink extra fluids after being burned.

2 cups (275 ml) boiled water

2 teaspoons (4 g) green tea leaves

2 teaspoons (4 g) chopped fresh spearmint

1 teaspoon (14 g) honey

2 tablespoons (28 ml) fresh lime juice

PREPARATION AND USE:

Put the tea leaves in the boiled water to steep. Stir in the spearmint. Continue to steep for 15 minutes. Strain the tea and stir in the honey until dissolved. Chill the remaining liquid. Stir in the lime juice and serve.

YIELD: 1 application

❓ **How it works:** As noted earlier, science touts green tea for its antibacterial, antioxidant, and anti-inflammatory properties. Although it can be topically applied to help guard skin from the sun's damaging rays, consuming green tea also helps provide protection against the detrimental effects of ultraviolet light.

WHEN SIMPLE DOESN'T WORK

- Take acetaminophen (Tylenol), ibuprofen (Motrin, Advil), or naproxen (Aleve, Naprosyn) for pain.
- Over-the-counter anesthetic creams and sprays can reduce discomfort.

Burn-out (Delicious Roasted) Chicken

Your body needs extra protein to heal wounds. Unless the burned area is small, be sure to consume enough during the process.

1 teaspoon (1 g) freshly ground black pepper

½ teaspoon sea salt

¼ cup (7 g) crushed fresh rosemary

1 whole chicken, (4 pounds, or 1.8 kg),
thoroughly washed, with skin

2 sprigs of rosemary

PREPARATION AND USE:

Preheat the oven to 350°F (180°C, or gas mark 4). Crush together the pepper, salt, and rosemary. Lifting up the chicken skin, rub the dry mixture directly onto the flesh. Re-cover the chicken with the skin. Place the rosemary sprigs inside the chicken cavity. Place the chicken on a rack in a baking pan. Roast uncovered for 20 minutes per pound, plus an extra 15 minutes. A meat thermometer should read 165°F (74°C). Remove from the oven and cover with aluminum foil for about 10 minutes. Slice and serve.

YIELD:6 servings

❓ How it works: When you have a wound of significant size, your body needs extra protein for healing. Chicken—white and dark meat—provides ample protein. When you've plucked the bones clean, use them to make delicious bone soup.

Colds

Few people make it through the winter without the familiar symptoms—sniffles, sneezes, and scratchy throat. The average adult catches two to four colds a year. Kids get at least twice that many colds. A chief reason is that the more than two hundred viruses that cause colds can survive on surfaces for hours. You push that grocery cart, borrow a pen, put away your kid's toys and then touch your finger to your nose or eyes, and—presto, you've inoculated yourself. Or someone sneezes or coughs a cloud of airborne viruses in your direction. Unless your immune system is in tip-top shape, symptoms follow in two to three days.

Fortunately, you have plenty of healing allies. And once you get sick, those pillars will support your recovery. Eat well. Unless you don't feel up to it, you can continue to exercise, which provides natural decongesting relief. Sleep is a great healer, though a stuffy nose can interfere. To reduce the risk of picking up other people's cold viruses or spreading yours to others, wash your hands often.

Although over-the-counter cold medications can decrease congestion, they don't cure the infection and may, in fact, prolong it. They can also create undesirable side effects. For instance, antihistamines dry and thicken secretions in your nose and elsewhere and make you feel even drowsier. To avoid a sinus infection, the goal is actually to thin respiratory mucus so it's easier to clear.

The good news is your kitchen holds a number of feel-better remedies. First, turn on the tap and drink a tall glass of cool water. Drink at least seven more glasses of warm liquids over the course of the day. Warm liquids are soothing, help increase blood circulation to the throat (and blood brings with it infection-fighting white blood cells), and speed clearance of respiratory mucus.

Next, put a kettle of water on to boil. Once it does, you have several options for recipes. You may want to try them all.

Throat Tonic

1 quart (946 ml) water

1 teaspoon (3 g) grated fresh ginger,
or ½ teaspoon dried

¼ cup (60 ml) fresh lemon juice

2 teaspoons (14 g) honey

PREPARATION AND USE:

Boil the water and then turn off the heat. Add the ginger. Cover and steep 20 minutes and then strain. Add the lemon juice and honey. Sip the quart of tonic over the course of the day. Reheat as necessary or drink at room temperature.

YIELD: 1 quart (946 ml) tonic

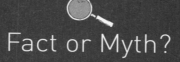

Fact or Myth?

BEING OUT IN THE COLD WILL CAUSE YOU TO CATCH COLD.

Studies show that's not true. However, being chilled stresses your body, and people who are under stress are more at risk for the common cold.

❓ How it works: The hot water is a hydrator that keeps your throat moist and also thins mucus and helps expel it. As you sip, simply breathing in the steam of the warm liquid helps with decongestion. Ginger is antimicrobial, antiinflammatory, analgesic, immune-enhancing, and an expectorant.

Congestion Clearance

1 quart (946 ml) water

2 to 3 drops eucalyptus essential oil

PREPARATION AND USE:

Boil the water and pour into a bowl. Add the eucalyptus essential oil. Cover your head with a clean towel. Lean over the bowl. Inhale through your nose to clear nasal congestion. (To clear lung congestion, inhale through your mouth.) Repeat three to five times a day as needed. Each time, you will need to reheat the water and add fresh plant essential oil. (Plant essential oils are volatile, meaning they vaporize quickly.)

YIELD: 1 steaming session

❓ How it works: Inhaling steam from the boiling water helps decongest nasal passages. (Breathe in slowly, as steam can burn your nose.) Oil of eucalyptus is an expectorant and antitussive (cough calming). It aids breathing by opening up bronchial tubes, easing congestion, and promoting sputum. It is also antimicrobial.

Note: If you have asthma, try using only steam first. If steam doesn't make you cough, add 1 drop of eucalyptus oil, working up to 3 drops as tolerated. In some people with asthma, inhaling the vapors from plant essential oils may trigger coughing.

Cold Crusher

Linda's former student Gina Penka, a childbirth educator, swears by this remedy. This recipe is best prepared at least one week in advance.

1 head garlic, cloves peeled and crushed

1 medium-size horseradish root, peeled
and coarsely chopped

1 finger-size slice of ginger, peeled and coarsely chopped

Apple cider vinegar

PREPARATION AND USE:

Place the crushed garlic cloves, horseradish root, and ginger in a clean, pint-size (475 ml) jar. Cover with apple cider vinegar until the fluid level clears the chopped ingredients by 1 inch (2.5 cm). Close the lid snugly. Shake.

Store in a covered cabinet. After two weeks, the chemicals in the plants will have largely moved into the vinegar. You now have two options. One is to strain and rebottle the vinegar extract and store it in the refrigerator. The second (Gina's preferred method) is to leave the herbs in the jar and eat them with the vinegar extraction.

Sip 1 to 2 tablespoons (15 to 30 ml) of this mixture at the first sign of cold symptoms. You can dilute the vinegar with herb tea or warm water. If you're feeling brave, chew a piece of garlic clove. Repeat each day for the first three days of the cold.

❓ How it works: There is evidence that garlic stimulates the immune system and may defend against catching a cold. It may also help fight viruses. In one study, participants who took garlic supplements for twelve weeks during the winter experienced a significant reduction in colds and a reduction in the symptoms of those colds that did occur. Ginger is antibacterial, anti-inflammatory, immune-enhancing, and calms coughing. Onions, which are botanical cousins of garlic, are also immune-enhancing, anti-inflammatory, and antimicrobial. The spiciness of horseradish stimulates thin nasal secretions, which helps clear away viruses.

Fact or Myth?

VITAMIN C PREVENTS THE COMMON COLD.

It is hard to say. Some studies show success, but many do not. Vitamin C supplements may be effective in people subjected to physical stress, such as performing vigorous exercise in very cold weather.

Echinacea Tincture

Tinctures made with plant extracts, water, and ethanol (alcohol) are
surprisingly simple to make. Vodka has the right blend of water and ethanol.

1 cup (26 g) ground echinacea root (*Echinacea purpurea*)

1½ cups (355 ml) vodka

PREPARATION AND USE:

Most echinacea root sold in natural food stores, herb stores, and online
comes in small chunks. Grind it in a food mill or clean coffee grinder. Pour
the ground root into a pint-size (475 ml) jar. Cover with vodka. Stir with
a chopstick or other small stirring device. Add more vodka, to the point
at which a good inch (2.5 cm) of liquid stands above the level of the herb.
Cover tightly and shake vigorously.

Store in a cabinet, shaking daily, for at least two weeks. (If you can wait four
to six weeks, great. Otherwise, you're ready to strain.) Wash and dry your
hands. Place a strainer over a bowl or large glass measuring cup. Lay
a square of cheesecloth or muslin over the strainer. Pour the tincture
through the cheesecloth, using a spoon to scrape out all the root. Wrap the
cheesecloth around the wet root and wring as much liquid as you can from
the plant. Compost the spent herb. Pour the tincture into a clean, dry pint-
size jar. Cap and store in the cupboard. It will keep for years.

At the first sign of cold symptoms, take ½ teaspoon of the tincture mixed
with water or tea every 2 hours while awake. After two days, reduce the
dosage to ½ teaspoon three times a day for the duration of the cold.

YIELD: About 48 doses

? How it works: Echinacea enhances immune function and has antiviral effects against respiratory viruses. The majority of studies on echinacea show that the herb modestly reduces cold severity and duration. The reduction is only about 10 to 30 percent.

The key to success is that a good product (the fresh juice of *E. purpurea* preserved in alcohol or root extracts from *E. purpurea* and *E. angustifolia*) must be taken frequently. Ground, encapsulated herb doesn't work. Infrequent dosing doesn't work, either. One study did show success when people drank five to six cups (1.2 to 1.4 L) per day of an echinacea tea.

! Warning: Echinacea is in the same plant family as ragweed. Some people are allergic to it. If you develop any symptoms of allergy, discontinue use.

Constipation

What is the most common digestive complaint in the United States? Constipation. We probably don't need to explain the symptoms, but forgive us for stating the obvious. Stools become hard, dry, and sometimes painful to pass. Although frequency usually declines, irregularity is not the defining characteristic. Not everyone has a daily bowel movement. Constipation is more common in seniors and affects women three times more often more than it does men. If constipation persists more than three months, it's considered chronic.

With advancing age, intestinal motility slows, allowing more time for water to be absorbed into the circulation, which leads to harder stools. Constipation and alternating constipation and diarrhea occur in irritable bowel syndrome, a condition of altered motility of the large intestine. Constipation is a common sign of hypothyroidism. Less often, the large intestine becomes obstructed. Damage to local nerves is another cause. Rare congenital conditions can also come with the absence of bowel movements.

In addition to making you uncomfortable, constipation has other negative consequences. Passage of hard stools may tear the anus, resulting in a vicious cycle where reluctance to re-experience the pain worsens constipation. Children going through toilet training are particularly vulnerable to that scenario.

Repeatedly straining to defecate can lead to hemorrhoids, varicose veins in the legs, and *diverticulosis* (a condition wherein small pouches protrude from the wall of the large intestine). In women, constipation contributes to pelvic floor prolapse (the descent of pelvic organs). In short, it's important to correct the condition.

RECItES TO TREAT CONSTIPATION

Psyllium Seed Husk Elixir

½ cup (120 ml) 100 percent apple juice

1½ cups (355 ml) water, divided

1 to 2 teaspoons (6 to 12 g) psyllium husks

PREPARATION AND USE:

Mix the apple juice and ½ cup (60 ml) of the water in a glass. Stir in the psyllium and drink the remaining water. Take two to three times a day.

YIELD: 1 serving

❓ **How it works:** Apple juice has a laxative effect. Both black and blond psyllium husks act as bulk-forming laxatives, which means their fiber holds water in the intestine, making the stool softer and easier to pass. Studies show that psyllium can be more effective than over-the-counter stool softeners, such as Colace (docusate sodium).

Note: Be sure to chase a glass of a psyllium beverage with an additional tall glass of water. Fiber doesn't help unless you consume water with it. In fact, insufficient water used with such products as Metamucil (whose active ingredient is psyllium husks) can make constipation worse.

A "Regular" Smoothie

This is easy—and effective! The flaxseeds and psyllium are a strong regulating combo. Instead of using an ice cube, try freezing the fruit in advance for a full, smooth texture.

½ banana

1½ teaspoons (11 g) flaxseed meal

1 teaspoon (6 g) psyllium husks

¾ cup (109 g) strawberries or (190 g) raspberries

½ cup (120 ml) almond milk

PREPARATION AND USE:

Place all the ingredients in a blender and blend well. Grind in an ice cube for a frothy finish.

YIELD: 1 serving

❓ **How it works:** The fiber in psyllium and fruit help soften the stool. Flaxseed meal adds omega-3 fatty acids, which provide antioxidant and anti-inflammatory action. Flaxseeds also ought to act as a bulk-forming laxative, but research confirmation is lacking.

Bean Soup Delight

A cold winter day, navy bean soup simmering on the stove, and a regulated system: all equal delight.

1 tablespoon (15 ml) canola oil

1 slice bacon (turkey or vegetarian), chopped into small bits

1 cup (160 g) chopped onion

½ cup (50 g) chopped celery

2 cans (15 ounces, or 428 g) navy beans, drained and rinsed

1 cup (235 ml) low-sodium vegetable or
chicken stock

¼ teaspoon sea salt

¼ cup (85 g) honey

PREPARATION AND USE:

Place the oil and bacon bits in a large pot over medium heat and sauté for about 2 minutes. Drop in the onion and celery and sauté until the onion becomes transparent, 3 to 5 minutes. Add the beans and stir well. Pour in the stock and bring to a boil. Stir in the sea salt and honey. Lower the heat and simmer for about 15 minutes, until the beans are tender. Serve.

YIELD: 4 servings

❓ **How it works:** Navy beans provide twice as much fiber as most vegetables—a whopping 9.5 grams in just ½ cup (91 g). They play a strong part in reversing constipation.

Johnny Apple Treat

John Chapman, my distant cousin, was the infamous Johnny Appleseed—no joke! He spread the word that apples had medicinal qualities. They are delicious, while effective, especially for constipation. ~ BBG

1 apple

¼ cup (35 g) raisins

¼ cup (30 g) chopped walnuts

1 tablespoon (15 g) fresh lemon juice

PREPARATION AND USE:

Coarsely grate the apple into a small bowl. Mix in the walnuts and raisins. Add the lemon juice and toss. Sprinkle with cinnamon to taste and enjoy.

YIELD: 2 servings

❓ **How it works:** Fresh apples are high in fiber, which adds bulk to the stool. They contain both soluble and insoluble fiber, also called roughage.

Super Greens with Olive Oil–Lemon Dressing

Enjoy this refreshing mix of greens—the lemon dressing adds to the zesty yet smooth flavor.

For the salad:

1 cup (20 g) arugula

1 cup (47 g) romaine lettuce

½ cup (25 g) sprouts

1 cup (40 g) torn fresh basil leaves, loosely packed

2 scallions, diced

1 avocado, peeled, pitted, and cut into chunks

For the dressing:

2 teaspoons (6 g) minced garlic

1 teaspoon (6 g) sea salt

2 tablespoons (30 ml) olive oil

2 tablespoons (30 ml) fresh lemon juice

¼ cup (30 g) dried cranberries

Freshly ground black pepper, to taste

PREPARATION AND USE:

To make the salad: Wash and drain the arugula, romaine, sprouts, and basil leaves. Toss together in a large bowl. Mix in the scallions and avocado chunks.

To make the dressing: In a small bowl, mash together the garlic and sea salt to form a paste. In another bowl, whisk together the lemon juice and olive oil and pour into a clean jar. Add the garlic paste to the jar. Close tightly and shake rapidly until combined.

Pour the dressing over the salad and sprinkle with the cranberries. Add pepper and toss.

YIELD: 4 servings

❓ **How it works:** Olive oil has a mild laxative effect. The greens in this salad provide fiber.

Note: Vary this recipe to use your favorite greens or just use one super green at a time! (The leftover dressing makes an excellent marinade.)

Cantaloupe with Honey-Yogurt Dressing

1 cup (230 g) plain yogurt
1 tablespoon (20 g) honey
½ teaspoon ground cinnamon
1 cantaloupe, seeded and cut into bite-size chunks

PREPARATION AND USE:

In a small bowl, blend together the yogurt, honey, and cinnamon. Portion the cantaloupe among 6 small bowls. Drizzle the honey-yogurt dressing over each serving.

YIELD: 6 servings

❓ **How it works:** Yogurt contains probiotics, living bacteria with health benefits, which promote intestinal health. Several studies have shown that fermented dairy products (fermented milk, in most cases) improve childhood constipation. Probiotic mixtures have been shown to relieve constipation in pregnant women, too. Cantaloupe contains fiber and magnesium.

Coughs

— and —

Bronchitis

Coughing is the symptom that most often sends people to their doctors. Anything that irritates the airways—infection, tobacco smoke, other air pollutants, allergens, an inhaled foreign object—causes coughing. It's one of the body's defenses against illness. In fact, elderly or otherwise debilitated people are more at risk for pneumonia because they can't summon a forceful, airway-clearing cough.

The most common cause of cough is acute bronchitis. Ninety percent of the time, the infectious agent is a virus. Typically, symptoms start in the upper airways with a sore throat and runny nose. Some viruses are more likely to extend below the trachea (windpipe) into the bronchi (large airways that deliver oxygen to the lung's tiny air sacs). The mucous membranes lining the bronchi swell and generate more mucus. Cilia, tiny hairlike projections from the cell that normally move the mucus carpet upward toward the mouth, become paralyzed. The cough normally lasts three weeks, longer after a bout of influenza. Expectoration of yellowish phlegm is normal and indicates your immune system is doing its work.

Other causes of coughs: Allergic rhinitis (hay fever) and sinusitis can lead to postnasal drip, which tends to produce a nighttime cough. Gastroesophageal reflux disease (GERD, or heartburn) can cause coughing and sometimes a burning sensation. Colds can aggravate asthma, which can produce coughing, and more easily lead to bronchitis. People with cystic fibrosis are very vulnerable to lung infections.

Chronic bronchitis (cough lasting longer than three months) is common in smokers and those who live with them. Tobacco smoke compromises immune defenses, inflames the bronchial linings, increases mucus, and paralyzes the cilia. People with chronic bronchitis are more at risk of acute infection.

Garlic Honey

4 garlic heads

1½ cups (480 g) honey

PREPARATION AND USE:

Peel the cloves and gently squash each one with the flat of the knife.
(Doing so activates an enzyme that converts an inactive chemical in garlic
to one of the key ingredients.) Drop the cloves into a clean pint-size (475
ml) mason jar. Add enough honey to completely cover the garlic. Stir with
a chopstick. Cap the jar. Let it sit for four to six weeks in a cool, dry place.
(If you already have a cough, you can dip into the honey pot in two days.)
You can eat the garlic cloves along with the honey.

YIELD: About 50 doses

❓ How it works: Honey is antibacterial and moistening. Studies show
that honey reduces nighttime cough in children more effectively than a
placebo, antihistamines, and the cough suppressant dextromethorphan.
Garlic is antimicrobial and an expectorant. Some of its chemicals are
excreted across the lungs. Although that may give you garlic breath, the
good news is some of garlic's beneficial chemicals are coming into contact
with your lungs.

Old Thyme-y Honey

½ cup (43 g) dried thyme leaves or (38 g) fresh

1½ to 2 cups (480 to 640 g) honey

PREPARATION AND USE:

You have two choices for prep:

1. Pour the thyme into a clean pint-size (475 ml) mason jar. Cover completely with honey. Stir to blend (a chopstick works well for stirring). Let sit for two weeks in a sunny window. At this point, you can either call the recipe done or strain the honey, discard the herbs, and rebottle. We don't mind the thyme leaves and hate to waste the delicious honey clinging to the leaves. Store in the cupboard.

2. Put the thyme in the top of a double boiler. Add enough honey to completely cover it. Add water to the bottom pan and bring to a boil. Lower the heat to a simmer. Keeping an eye on the honey, and stirring frequently, simmer for 2 hours. You can either bottle it with the thyme leaves or strain out the thyme leaves and bottle the herb-infused honey. Take honey by the teaspoon to relieve coughing.

YIELD: About 24 doses (less if the thyme is removed, more if it isn't)

❓ **How it works:** Thyme helps open tight airways, combats infection, calms coughs, and helps expel mucus.

Peppermint Honey

¼ cup (80 g) honey

3 to 5 drops peppermint essential oil

PREPARATION AND USE:

Put the honey and peppermint essential oil in a small, clean jar and blend with a chopstick. Cap and store in a cupboard. Take 1 teaspoonful up to four times a day.

YIELD: 12 doses

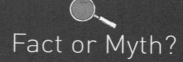

Fact or Myth?

FOR ANY AGE, OVER-THE-COUNTER REMEDIES ARE THE QUICKEST, STRONGEST COUGH RELIEVERS.

Myth. Research indicates they're not effective in kids under six years old and carry significant risks. In fact, they are downright dangerous for kids under the age of two. In adults, expectorants don't improve outcomes. Cough suppressants, however, can make sense for teens and adults when coughing interferes with sleep. (You can't cough and sleep at the same time. Each coughing episode wakes you.)

❓ How it works: Peppermint reduces chest tightness and coughing and helps clear mucus.

❗ Warning: This recipe is for teens and adults only. Most of the time, essential oils are used externally only. However, peppermint is safe in small amounts.

Italian Steam

2 cups (475 ml) water

½ cup (about 24 g) Italian seasonings: fresh thyme, oregano, and/or rosemary leaves

PREPARATION AND USE:

Boil the water in a saucepan. Turn off the heat. Add a handful of the herbs and stir. Cover for 10 minutes. Remove from the heat and set on a hot pad. Remove the lid. Lean over the steaming water and cover your head with a clean towel. Breathe the vapors through your mouth for about 1 minute. Rewarm and repeat several times a day as needed. If you store the covered saucepan overnight in the refrigerator, you may reuse the next day.

YIELD: One to two days' worth of steaming

❓ How it works: These Italian seasonings are all members of the peppermint family. As such, they relax smooth muscle (thus relaxing the airways) and discourage infection.

Note: If you have eucalyptus trees in your area, you can substitute those leaves, crushed, for the Italian herbs.

Eucalyptus Steam

2 cups (475 ml) water

2 to 3 drops eucalyptus essential oil

PREPARATION AND USE:

Boil the water in a saucepan. Turn off the heat. Transfer the pan to a hot pad. Add 2 to 3 drops of eucalyptus oil. Bend over the pan and cover your head with a clean towel. Inhale the steam through your mouth for about 1 minute. Repeat four or five times a day. Because the essential oil vaporizes quickly, you'll need to reheat the water and add fresh eucalyptus essential oil each time.

YIELD: 1 steam session

❓ **How it works:** Essential oil of eucalyptus works against a range of bacteria and viruses. It also favorably alters immune function and helps clear excess respiratory mucus. By breathing in through your mouth, you allow the essential oil steam to come in direct contact with your throat.

Note: Inhaling vapors from the smell of essential oils may trigger asthmatic coughing. If you have asthma, try plain steam first. If the steam doesn't trigger your asthma or worsen your coughing, add 1 drop of essential oil. If you tolerate that, work your way up to three. People with asthma usually have no problem using chest rubs that include essential oils, such as eucalyptus.

Cough-Cutting Peppermint Tea

2 cups (475 ml) water

1 teaspoon (1 g) dried thyme

3 teaspoons (5 g) dried peppermint leaves

Honey (optional)

PREPARATION AND USE:

Bring the water to a boil in a small pan. Add the herbs. Remove the pan from the heat. Cover and steep for 15 minutes. Strain and add honey, if desired. Drink the tea and inhale the steam through your mouth. Try to drink several cups a day.

YIELD: 1 serving

❓ How it works: Peppermint and thyme both help calm coughs and combat infection. Peppermint can also ease throat discomfort associated with coughing.

Note: Buy a box of peppermint tea bags and keep them handy for your this remedy.

Lemon Up

1 lemon

Less than $\frac{1}{8}$ teaspoon freshly ground black pepper

PREPARATION AND USE:

Slice the lemon in half. Sprinkle the black pepper over one half. Suck in the liquid and swallow. Brush your teeth afterward to remove the acidity from your teeth.

YIELD: 1 serving

❓ **How it works:** Lemon packs flavonoids and vitamin C for fighting infection. Pepper increases circulation, which helps the healing process.

Mustard Plaster

Ask someone to assist you with the application of this remedy.

1 tablespoon (9 g) dry mustard

1 tablespoon (8 g) all-purpose flour

1 tablespoon (15 ml) warm water, plus more as needed

1 tablespoon (15 ml) olive oil

PREPARATION AND USE:

Mix the mustard and flour in a small bowl. Blend in the water. Add more water as needed to make a spreadable paste. Cover your chest with the olive oil (it will protect the skin from mustard's somewhat irritating effects). Place a clean cloth on your chest (use a bandana, thin dishcloth, or muslin—something you don't mind turning yellow). Spread the mustard plaster over the cloth. Cover the plaster with a plastic bag.

On top, place a warm, moist hand towel (your assistant can heat it in the microwave on high for 30 to 60 seconds). After 5 minutes, remove the mustard plaster and wash your skin. Do not leave on longer, as blistering can occur.

YIELD: 1 application

❓ **How it works:** Mustard contains irritating chemicals that stimulate blood flow. The idea is that increasing blood supply promotes delivery of infection-fighting white blood cells. While the infection isn't in the skin, this plaster can create a deeper sense of warmth. This traditional remedy has not, as far as we know, been subjected to scientific study. However, many people swear by this remedy.

Note: If you have sensitive skin or allergies, try a small test patch first. Cases of contact dermatitis (allergic skin reactions) have been reported. Do not apply to inflamed skin or open wounds.

WHEN SIMPLE DOESN'T WORK

Several studies support the use of an extract of pelargonium (*Pelargonium sidoides*, a South African geranium) as a bronchitis treatment. The Zulu have long used this plant. In one study, people taking it returned to work two days sooner than did those taking a placebo. You can find this product in natural food stores sold under the brand name Umcka.

Diarrhea

A long list of maladies can cause diarrhea. Infections are a common cause of acute diarrhea. Accompanying symptoms often include nausea, vomiting, mild fever, cramping, and general malaise. Microbes infecting the gastrointestinal tract include viruses (rotavirus and Norwalk virus), bacteria (*E. coli*, *Salmonella*, *Shigella*, *Campylobacter*, and *Vibrio cholerae*), and protozoa (giardia and amoebas). Toxins produced by bacteria also make us sick.

Food allergies and intolerances (e.g., lactose intolerance) can cause gas, crampy pain, diarrhea, and vomiting. Allergic foods also cause hives and swelling of respiratory linings.

Food poisoning and consumption of poisonous foods (e.g., poisonous mushrooms) usually also cause vomiting. Antibiotics disrupt the normal microbial ecosystem to cause diarrhea. Overconsumption of fruit and fruit juice loosens stools. Fear and extreme anxiety can trigger a precipitous emptying of the bowels.

Some chronic conditions are associated with recurrent diarrhea. In irritable bowel syndrome (also called spastic colon), a condition of altered bowel motility, diarrhea may alternate with constipation. Inflammatory bowel diseases, which include Crohn's disease and ulcerative colitis, result in recurrent diarrhea (which may contain blood or pus), fatigue, fever, abdominal pain, and trouble maintaining weight. In celiac disease, consumption of gluten (a protein in certain grains) leads to an immune system attack on the intestinal lining. Hyperthyroidism speeds bowel activity, which means there isn't enough time for water to be absorbed into the blood.

Chronic conditions require careful medical management. If allergies or intolerance upset your stomach, avoid those foods. Allergy testing, careful food diaries, and elimination diets (removing all potential culprits for several days, then slowly reintroducing them one at a time) can help pinpoint the offending foods.

Food poisoning and infectious gastroenteritis (inflammation of the stomach and intestines) usually resolve within twenty-four to seventy-two hours. During that time, it's important to rest and replace fluid losses with clear liquids—but not simply water. You also need salt and sugar. Steer clear of apple juice and prune juice, which loosen stools. Because you may temporarily lose the ability to digest dairy, skip that food group until several days after you recover. The foods you eat should be bland, relatively low in fiber, and easy to digest. This chapter offers some recipes you can try.

Green Tea, Lemon, and Honey

1 cup (235 ml) water

2 teaspoons (4 g) loose green tea

1 teaspoon (7 g) honey

1 teaspoon (5 ml) fresh lemon juice

PREPARATION AND USE:

In a saucepan, boil the water and add the tea. Turn off the heat, cover, and steep for 1 to 3 minutes. In a cup, mix the honey and lemon juice. Strain out the tea leaves and pour the tea into the honey mixture.

YIELD: 1 serving

❓ How it works: Green tea is astringent and it inhibits major food-borne bacteria, such as *E. coli*, *Salmonella typhimurium*, and *Staphylococcus* aureus. Lemon is astringent, too, and contains vitamin C and bioflavonoids, which support the immune system. The essential oils in citrus fruits also discourage bacteria such as *E. coli* and *Salmonella*. Honey is anti-inflammatory, soothing, immune system–enhancing, and antibacterial.

Moderating Miso

¼ cup (64 g) miso paste

2 cups (475 ml) water

1 scallion, chopped

2 garlic cloves, minced

PREPARATION AND USE:

Spoon the miso paste into a bowl. Boil the water in a saucepan and lower the heat to low. Pour ¼ cup (60 ml) of boiled water into the bowl with the miso, and stir until the mixture is smooth. mAdd the miso mixture to the remaining water in the saucepan. Stir until fully blended. Add the scallion. Stir in the garlic just before serving (by not cooking the garlic, you maintain it's key ingredients).

YIELD: 2 servings

❓ **How it works:** Miso, which is made from fermented soybeans, contains probiotics. In research showing that probiotics shorten the course of diarrhea, volunteers received supplemental bacteria. Scientists have not yet studied miso as a remedy for diarrhea. But it will help correct loss of salty and alkaline fluid. Raw garlic inhibits a number of bacteria, viruses, protozoa, and worms.

The Big Apple—Sauced

½ cup (120 ml) water

2 unpeeled apples, cored and cut into chunks

¼ teaspoon ground cinnamon

1 tablespoon (20 g) honey

PREPARATION AND USE:

Pour the water into a saucepan. Add the apples, cinnamon, and honey and stir together. Cook the mixture over medium heat for about 15 minutes or until the apples are soft. Let the apple mixture cool and mash with a fork.

YIELD: 3 to 4 servings

❓ **How it works:** Apples, particularly the peels, contain pectin. If you've ever made jam, you known that pectin draws water to make a gel. In that way, it reduces watery diarrhea. Because raw apples are harder to digest, it's better to consume cooked apples. If you don't feel up to cooking, use store-bought applesauce. Cinnamon contains the antibacterial agent cinnamaldehyde. Honey is anti-inflammatory, soothing, and inhibits some bacterial species.

Skinny Oats

½ cup (40 g) rolled oats

1 cup (235 ml) water

½ teaspoon ground cinnamon

1 teaspoon (14 g) honey (optional)

PREPARATION AND USE:

Mix together the oats, water, and cinnamon in a microwave-safe dish. Heat on high for 3 minutes. (Alternatively, combine the oats and cinnamon in a dish or measuring cup. Boil the water in a small pan, and then stir in the oats and cinnamon. Lower the heat to medium-low and cook, stirring occasionally, for 5 to 8 minutes until the oats reach your desired consistency.) Add the honey, if desired. Let cool and eat.

YIELD: 1 to 2 servings

❓ How it works: Oats are soothing to irritated linings and contain a complex carbohydrate that enhances immune function. Honey has anti-inflammatory and antibacterial properties. Cinnamon is antibacterial.

Carob Shake

2 small or 1 large banana, chopped

½ cup (65 g) raspberries (optional)

½ cup (115 g) plain yogurt (Read the label

to buy a yogurt with probiotic organisms.)

1 tablespoon (6.5 g) carob powder

1 tablespoon (20 g) honey

PREPARATION AND USE:

Combine the bananas and raspberries, if using, in a blender and blend until smooth. Add the yogurt, carob powder, and honey and fully blend. Serve.

YIELD: 1 serving

? **How it works:** Carob (locust bean) contains locust bean gum, a polysaccharide that binds water. Tannins in carob have an astringent effect. Bananas are a bland, soothing food. They provide needed sugars and potassium. The probiotics, or good bacteria, in some yogurts can help relieve infectious diarrhea—the kind encountered by travelers—by fighting the bad bacteria in the intestines. Whereas many dairy products are difficult to digest during a bout of infectious diarrhea, yogurt can often be tolerated.

Soothing Carrot-Ginger Soup

2 cups (475 ml) water

1 cup (130 g) scrubbed, chopped carrot

2 tablespoons (28 g) unsalted butter

1 teaspoon (7 g) honey (optional)

½ tablespoon fresh lemon juice

¼ teaspoon ground ginger

1 vegetable bouillon cube

PREPARATION AND USE:

Bring the water to a boil in a saucepan. Add the carrot and cook about 7 minutes until tender. Meanwhile, melt the butter in a skillet over low heat and stir in the honey, if using. Mix together the lemon juice and ginger in the skillet. Strain the carrots, reserving the liquid, and stir into the skillet mixture. Pour the carrot cooking liquid back into saucepan and add the bouillon cube. Add the skillet mixture to the saucepan and cover. Simmer for about 5 minutes.

YIELD: 2 servings

❓ How it works: Carrot soup and carrot juice are traditional remedies for diarrhea. Carrots are rich in a number of vitamins, many of which support immune health, and also minerals, including potassium, which diarrhea depletes. They also supply sugars. Cooked carrots are easier to digest than raw. Ginger is antibacterial and eases upset stomachs.

Rehydration Drink

For the first day, stick to clear liquids. This is a variant of the recipe on page 121, adapted from the Rehydration Project. This nonprofit international group works to curb the high death rate of children in developing countries from infections.

¼ cup (60 ml) fresh orange juice

2 cups (475 ml) room-temperature water

¼ teaspoon baking soda

2 teaspoons (14 g) honey

PREPARATION AND USE:

Combine the orange juice and water in a small pitcher. Stir in the baking soda until dissolved. Stir in the honey until dissolved.

YIELD: 2 servings

❓ **How it works:** The biggest risk associated with diarrhea is dehydration. Children and the elderly are most vulnerable. This drink replaces depleted water, salt, potassium, and sugar. The baking soda also helps correct losses of alkaline fluid.

Blackberry Tea

If you have access to blackberry (or raspberry) leaves or roots, this time-honored recipe can help slow the flow.

3 cups (710 ml) water
2 tablespoons (3 g) chopped dried
blackberry leaves, or 4 tablespoons
(24 g) fresh honey

PREPARATION AND USE:
Boil the water. Add the leaves. Turn off the heat, cover, and steep for 15 to 20 minutes. (If you also add blackberry roots, turn the heat to low and simmer for 20 minutes.) Strain. Sweeten with honey, to taste.

YIELD: 3 servings

❓ How it works: Blackberry tea is an astringent, which gently contracts and helps dry tissues in the intestinal tract.

Hay Fever

— and —

Seasonal Allergies

For many people, spring is the sneezin' season. Other symptoms of hay fever (allergic rhinitis in the medical world) include nasal congestion and itchy and watery nose and eyes. If you only have these symptoms a couple of months, consider yourself lucky. Some people have a year-round condition called perennial rhinitis. Triggers include pollen, molds, dust mites, animal dander, and other airborne offenders.

llergic and perennial rhinitis tends to run in families, along with asthma nd atopic dermatitis (eczema). In recent decades, the prevalence of all hree conditions has risen. A warmer climate with longer growing seasons s expected to increase the pollen load for hay fever sufferers.

he underlying problem is immune system hypersensitivity. The immune ystem detects a speck of ragweed pollen and reacts as though an army f streptococci had invaded. In response, white blood cells produce a type f antibody called immunoglobulin E (IgE), which binds to mast cells, mmune system cells involved in allergic reactions. Once IgE binds to mast ells, the latter release histamine and other inflammatory chemicals that ause those well-known symptoms.

Conventional treatment calls for avoiding known allergens and aking medication, such as antihistamines, to reduce symptoms. Side effects include excessive drying of the mouth, nose, and throat. The older antihistamines, such as diphenhydramine (Benadryl) and chlorpheniramine, also cause drowsiness. Newer antihistamines, such as loratadine (Claritin) and fexofenadine (Allegra), are less sedating. Intranasal steroid sprays and other medications can manage symptoms in people with persistent symptoms. Finally, immunotherapy ("allergy shots") may be used to desensitize people to allergens (the substance that causes an allergic reaction).

Blushing Apple Smoothie

½ cup (78 g) pitted fresh cherries

½ English cucumber, peeled

1 apple, cored and peeled

½ cup (65 g) fresh raspberries

1 tablespoon (10 g) chia seeds

½ cup (120 ml) water

6 ice cubes

PREPARATION AND USE:

Place all the ingredients in a blender and blend until smooth.

YIELD: 3 servings

❓ **How it works:** Bioflavonoids, which are found in many fruits, vegetables, nuts, and seeds, are antioxidant, antihistamine, and inhibit histamine release. The fruits in this smoothie are rich in vitamin C, which blocks histamine release from mast cells. People with higher levels of vitamin C have lower levels of histamine. This vitamin also acts as an antioxidant and enhances immune function. Some but not all studies suggest vitamin C supplements can improve asthma and allergy.

Probiotic Salad

2 cups (340 g) sliced strawberries

1 cup (150 g) sliced red seedless grapes

1 apple, cored and sliced

1 celery stalk, sliced

¼ cup (35 g) raisins

½ cup (115 g) plain Greek yogurt

¼ cup (25 g) crushed almonds

Pinch of ground cinnamon

PREPARATION AND USE:

In a large bowl, mix the fresh fruits, raisins, and celery together. Fold in the yogurt. Chill for 30 minutes. Toss with the almonds and serve with a pinch of cinnamon.

YIELD: 2 servings

❓ How it works: People with a genetic predisposition to asthma, allergic rhinitis, and eczema have a different microbial ecosystem in their intestines than allergy-free people do. Yogurt contains live, health-promoting microbes (probiotics) that benefit immune health. Supplemental probiotics have been shown to reduce certain allergic symptoms in children.

Chia Breakfast Pudding

2 cups (475 ml) almond milk

5 tablespoons (59 g) chia seeds

1 banana, sliced

2 teaspoons (14 g) honey

Ground cinnamon

PREPARATION AND USE:

In a saucepan, heat the milk to just before boiling; do not boil. Stir in the chia seeds. Remove from the heat and let stand for about 10 minutes, stirring a few times, until the mixture begins to gel. Reheat the mixture until it is your desired warmth. Divide between two dishes and top each with ½ banana, 1 teaspoon (7 g) of honey, and a sprinkle of cinnamon.

YIELD: 2 servings

How it works: Chia seeds (also hemp seeds and flaxseeds) contain omega-3 fatty acids, which are anti-inflammatory. In addition to consuming more of these healthful fats, we recommend you reduce intake of foods that contain fats that increase inflammation, such as meat and processed foods. A study in pregnant Japanese women showed that eating more meat correlated with more symptoms such as watery eyes and nose. On the other hand, greater consumption of fish (a good source of omega-3 fats) correlated with less allergic rhinitis.

Honey-Sage Tea

Popular lore has it that local honey (made by bees visiting local plants) can reduce hay fever symptoms. New studies are confirming the benefits of honey.

2 cups (475 ml) water

2 teaspoons dried, crushed sage leaves

2 tablespoons (40 g) honey

PREPARATION AND USE:

In a small saucepan, bring the water to a boil. Add the sage. Turn off the heat. Cover and steep for 15 minutes. Stir in the honey. Sip and enjoy.

YIELD: 1 large or 2 small servings

❓ **How it works:** For nasal secretions, sage (Salvia officinalis) has a drying and anti-inflammatory effect. A Finnish study was able to confirm that, for people allergic to birch pollen, consuming steadily greater amounts of birch pollen honey between November and March (before hay fever season) had significantly fewer symptoms come spring. Do not give honey to infants under twelve months of age because of the small risk of botulism.

In-the-Bag Onion Soup

Leave the onion skins in a muslin bag in the soup until you serve it, so the antihistamine agent quercetin will have its strongest effect.

2 teaspoons (10 ml) olive oil

2 cups (320 g) thinly sliced sweet white or yellow onion, skins reserved

2 cups (320 g) thinly sliced red onion, skins reserved

2 teaspoons (6 g) minced fresh garlic

¼ teaspoon freshly ground black pepper

¼ teaspoon sugar, or ½ packet (1 g) stevia

2 tablespoons (30 ml) dry white wine

1 quart (946 ml) low-sodium vegetable stock

½ teaspoon chopped fresh thyme, or ¼ teaspoon dried

PREPARATION AND USE:

In a large saucepan, heat the olive oil over medium heat. Add the onion and sauté, stirring for 5 minutes. Add the garlic, pepper, and sugar and stir. Lower the heat. Continue to cook for another 20 minutes, adding small amounts of stock to keep moist. Meanwhile, place the reserved onion skins in a muslin bag.

Stir the wine into the pot and, after 1 minute, add the bag with the skins, remaining stock, and thyme. Lower the heat to low and simmer for 1 hour. Leave the onion skins in the broth until just before serving and then remove the muslin bag.

YIELD: 4 servings

? How it works: The skin and outer ring of onions contain the substance quercetin, which has an antihistamine effect. In a study of people with year-round allergic nasal symptoms, quercetin significantly inhibited histamine release. Furthermore, substances in onion called thiosulfinates seem to have anti-inflammatory activity and can inhibit bronchoconstriction (airway narrowing as occurs in asthma). Other foods with quercetin are grapefruit, red wine, apples, garlic, cayenne pepper, cabbage, and tea.

Fact or Myth?

A HUMIDIFIER WILL HELP SOOTHE YOUR ALLERGIES.

Yes and no. While moisture can soothe dry sinus passages, dust and mold can gather in the humidifier and actually do more harm than good. Clean and change the filter often and use distilled water. The high minerals in tap water encourage bacteria growth, which may cause further irritation.

Broiled Red Peppers

This is a specialty from the kitchen of Barbara Grogan's dear friend Sophia Eorio, who makes peppers, olive oil, and garlic a healthy part of her family's diet; her daughter Lisa whips up several batches ahead of time, and then makes divine roasted pepper sandwiches for drop-in lunch guests.

2 teaspoons (10 ml) olive oil

4 red bell peppers, cut in half, stemmed, and seeded

6 garlic cloves, sliced thinly

PREPARATION AND USE:

Preheat the oven to 450°F (230°C, or gas mark 8) and then turn it to broil. Spread a baking sheet with the olive oil. Cover with a layer of garlic and top with a layer of peppers. Place the baking sheet on the top rack of the oven. Broil for 15 to 20 minutes until the pepper skins blacken. Transfer the peppers and garlic to a platter and let cool, about 15 minutes. Place the peppers and garlic in a resealable plastic bag and store in the refrigerator. Remove the skins from the peppers (optional) and serve the roasted pepper and garlic in salads, sandwiches, soups, pastas, and more.

YIELD: 4 servings

❓ How it works: Studies link higher intake of beta-carotene with fewer allergies. Foods rich in beta-carotene include red peppers, romaine and other green and red-leaf lettuces, kale, carrots, spinach, dandelion greens (buy or pick in an area where pesticides haven't been used and where they have not been grown near the street), collards, cabbage, beet, mustard, and turnip greens, pumpkin, sweet potatoes, and winter squashes, such as butternut squash.

Note: Make sure to broil, not roast, the peppers. Roasting overcooks them.

Wakame Seaweed Salad

Juice of 2 honey tangerines or 1 Valencia orange

About ½ cup (10 g) dried wakame

2 tablespoons (30 ml) toasted sesame oil

A splash of hot sauce

2 tablespoons (16 g) sesame seeds

PREPARATION AND USE:

Place the tangerine juice into a bowl. Add enough seaweed to cover the juice. Let sit for about 20 minutes while the juice is absorbed. (Add more seaweed if the juice is not all absorbed.) Stir in the oil and hot sauce. Mix in the sesame seeds.

YIELD: 1 serving

❓ **How it works:** A Japanese dietary analysis of pregnant women found that seaweed stood out as protective against allergic rhinitis. Wakame, which is a type of seaweed, is rich in omega-3 fatty acids, vitamins, and minerals. It's also high in sodium; so take care if you're on a salt-restrictive diet.

Headaches: Migraine, Tension

— and —

Sinus

Headaches can be a miserable—and for some people, daily—experience. They come in different varieties, with tension headaches being the most common. Tight muscles in the neck, shoulders, and/or face create a viselike constriction. These headaches may evolve over the course of a taxing day.

In a condition called bruxism, people clench or grind their teeth, resulting in pain in the jaw and temples. Some people clench mainly at night and do so unwittingly. The main clue is morning face pain that subsides over the course of the day. Chewing gum or eating hard candy can aggravate the condition.

Migraines cause repeated episodes of intense, throbbing pain. The pain is usually localized to one side, centering on the temple, around the eye, or at the back of the head. About 20 percent of migraines are preceded by auras, which are marked by sensory distortion. Sensations are usually visual (blind spots in the vision, jagged lines, or flashing lights) but can also affect hearing, taste, and smell.

Cluster headaches, also called suicide headaches, center around one eye. Several headaches may occur in a single day. Or the cluster of headaches can stretch over a couple of months.

Medical treatment for headache includes nonsteroidal anti-inflammatory medicines, such as aspirin, acetaminophen, ibuprofen, and naproxen. People with migraines may take prescription medications such as the "triptans." Doctors typically prescribe medications taken daily to prevent frequent migraines.

People with what are called "frequent daily headaches" may get them due to a rebound effect from pain relievers. In other words, the medications create a vicious cycle.

Ginger-Feverfew Elixir

2 cups (235 ml) water

1 teaspoon (3 g) finely grated fresh ginger, packed

1 teaspoon (2 g) chopped fresh feverfew leaves, or ½ teaspoon dried

Honey or agave nectar

PREPARATION AND USE:

Bring the water to a boil. Add the ginger and simmer, uncovered, for 10 minutes. Remove from the heat and add the feverfew leaves. Cover and steep for 15 to 20 minutes. Strain out the ginger and feverfew. Stir in honey to taste, and serve hot.

YIELD: 2 servings

❓ How it works: Ginger reduces pain and inflammation. Its antinausea effect may help counteract nausea associated with migraines. Research indicates that feverfew extracts help prevent migraines, possibly due to anti-inflammatory effects and the prevention of the arterial constriction in the brain that contributes to these headaches. Fresh leaf extracts seem to work better than dried. Two studies have shown that special extracts combining ginger and feverfew can help to stop an evolving migraine.

Note: Feverfew is bitter; honey or agave will help the medicine go down.

Honey-Cinnamon Coffee

We used nondairy milk in this recipe because, for some people, allergies to cow's milk protein can trigger migraines. ~ LBW

1 cup (235 ml) freshly brewed coffee

¼ cup (60 ml) almond or other nondairy milk

¼ teaspoon vanilla extract

2 tablespoons (40 g) honey

¼ teaspoon ground cinnamon

PREPARATION AND USE:

In a saucepan, combine the coffee, nondairy milk, and vanilla. Warm until hot, but do not boil. Stir in the honey until dissolved. Stir in the cinnamon.

YIELD: About 2 servings

❓ How it works: Caffeine has a paradoxical effect on migraines. For people who consume it infrequently, it can help break a migraine. Scientists aren't sure exactly how it works, but point to mild analgesic action and effects upon blood vessel diameter and certain brain chemicals. Caffeine also increases the absorption of pain-relieving medications, which is why it's often combined with acetaminophen or aspirin for headache treatment. However, regular consumption of higher doses of caffeine (more than 300 milligrams, or about 3 cups [710 ml] of coffee a day) can contribute to the development of migraines. Withdrawal from caffeine can also make the head throb.

Bay Leaf Broth

1½ quarts (1.4 L) water

1 onion, diced

1 garlic clove, minced

⅛ teaspoon dried thyme

⅛ teaspoon dried rosemary

1 bay leaf

1 celery stalk, halved

⅛ teaspoon sea salt

Freshly ground black pepper

PREPARATION AND USE:

Stir together the water, onion, garlic, thyme, and rosemary in a pot. Add the bay leaf and celery. Bring to a boil. Lower the heat to low, cover, and simmer for 1 hour. (The longer you simmer the bay leaf, the more it infuses the broth with its healing properties.) Remove the bay leaf and celery. Season with salt and pepper to taste. Pour the steaming broth into mugs and enjoy.

YIELD: 6 servings

❓ **How it works:** Herbal experts, such as James Duke, Ph.D., recommend bay leaves for preventing migraines. The leaves contain some of the same chemicals as feverfew. Studies show that they block bodily chemicals that dilate arteries. (In migraines, exaggerated dilation of arteries painfully stretches nerves.) To date, no studies have investigated its use in preventing migraines.

Essential Oil Anti-Pain Massage

tablespoon (15 ml) carrier oil (try almond, apricot, or olive)

to 5 drops peppermint essential oil

PREPARATION AND USE:

Place the oils in a clean, small jar. Cover tightly with a lid. Shake until combined. Massage into sore areas: neck, shoulders, jaw, or temples. Take care not to touch your eyes. When finished, lie down in a quiet place with your eyes shut..

YIELD: 1 application

? How it works: Two studies show that peppermint essential oil, applied topically, helps relieve tension headaches. It seems to inhibit pain nerve receptors. In addition, massage is effective in relieving tightness in the tender neck, shoulder, and head muscles by increasing blood flow.

LIFESTYLE TIP

Don't skip meals—an empty stomach can trigger a migraine. Do eat a healthy, balanced diet low in fats. Doctors have seen a reduction in migraines when fats are reduced in the diet.

Essential Oil Pressure Point Relief

1 drop peppermint essential oil

1 drop lavender essential oil

PREPARATION AND USE:

Put a drop each of peppermint and lavender essential oil in one palm. Spread onto your fingers. Press your fingers into the muscles paralleling the spine between the base of your skull and your neck (about two finger widths on either side of your spine).

YIELD: 1 application

❓ **How it works:** As in the previous remedy, peppermint essential oil relieves headaches by inhibiting nerve receptors. Inhalation of lavender essential oil has also been shown to reduce migraine headache pain as well as nausea and sensitivity to light. Studies also show that this acupressure point and others can relieve pain in people with chronic headaches.

Hot Headache Relief

I use a commercial capsaicin ointment; this recipe naturally delivers capsaicin, the constituent of chile peppers that both creates heat and reduces pain. ~ LBW

2 teaspoons (10 ml) unscented hand cream

¼ teaspoon cayenne pepper

PREPARATION AND USE:

In a small, clean bowl, blend the hand cream and cayenne. Massage into your neck and shoulders.

YIELD: 1 application

How it works: Cayenne contains capsaicin, which interferes with the ability of nerves that transmit information about pain from the periphery to the brain. (Pain, though very real, is all in your head. If the brain doesn't get the news—well, what pain?) You can find over-the-counter ointments standardized for capsaicin in drugstores. Research suggests that special capsaicin preparations applied inside the nose (which we don't recommend you do with cayenne pepper or commercial ointments) can help block cluster headaches—severe, one-sided headaches that come in waves.

Warning: Do not touch your eyes when mixing or using this remedy. Also, this mixture could stain clothes. Expect to feel heat at the site of the application. Start with small amounts until you see how you respond.

Influenza

Influenza, or flu, is a highly contagious viral respiratory illness. In an average year, 5 to 20 percent of Americans will develop influenza, more than 200,000 will wind up in the hospital, and more than 36,000 will die. Those most vulnerable are people older than age sixty-five and younger than age two, as well as pregnant women and people with chronic medical conditions.

The virus spreads from person to person via respiratory droplets—tiny drops of moisture released into the air when an infected person talks, coughs, and sneezes. Bystanders may inhale the viruses through their mouths or nose. Flu viruses can also survive on inanimate objects for two to eight hours. If, after handling this object, you touch your eye, nose, or lip, you have inoculated yourself.

Signs and symptoms of influenza include sore throat, stuffy nose, cough, body aches, headache, fatigue, fever, and chills. Whereas the common cold mainly causes symptoms from the neck up, influenza causes more total-body misery. Also, coughing is more pronounced. Contagion begins the day before symptoms develop and extends for a week after symptoms begin. Most symptoms resolve within three to six days. However, fatigue and cough can linger for a few weeks.

Garlicky Honey

1 head garlic, cloves separated and peeled

2 thin slices onion

Honey

PREPARATION AND USE:

Using the flat of a knife, gently crush each clove—just enough to crack it open. Place the garlic cloves in a pint-size (475 ml) jar. Layer on the onion. Cover the garlic and onion with honey and cap the jar. Let the mixture sit in a warm place overnight. Take a spoonful of the honey to coat your throat; eating the garlic and onion will also provide relief. If you prefer not to eat the garlic and onion, you can strain the honey into a separate jar.

YIELD: Multiple servings

❓ **How it works:** Honey is soothing to inflamed respiratory passages and antibacterial (though the issue here is a viral infection). It's safer than over-the-counter cough remedies and at least as effective. Garlic is expectorant (helps clear respiratory mucus) and antimicrobial, including antiviral activity against influenza. Special extracts have been shown to decrease flu symptom severity. Onion is a close botanical relative of garlic and contains similar sulfur-containing compounds. It's antimicrobial and is used in folk medicine to clear respiratory mucus and open tight airways.

The D-Licious Fish

Three ounces (85 g) of salmon carry 794 IU of vitamin D, nearly the entire 1,000 IU a day recommended for the body to fight the respiratory upsets that accompany flu. Check the index for additional salmon recipes.

2 salmon steaks or fillets (3 ounces or 85 g)

2 teaspoons (10 ml) olive oil

Freshly ground black pepper

1 lemon, sliced

PREPARATION AND USE:

Preheat the oven to 375°F (190°C, or gas mark 5). Place a sheet of aluminum foil on a baking sheet. Place the salmon on the foil (if using fillets, place skin side down) and baste with the olive oil. Rub in the ground pepper. Cover each steak with the lemon slices. Fold the foil into a tent over the fish. Bake for about 20 minutes until the fish just flakes with a fork. Serve.

YIELD: 2 servings

❓ How it works: Salmon is a go-to food for vitamin D; it also contains anti-inflammatory fatty acids. Vitamin D also helps the immune system function optimally. Many people have suboptimal blood levels of this vitamin. Several studies have linked low levels of vitamin D with a higher risk for respiratory infection. Some studies further suggest that dietary supplementation may lower the risk of respiratory infection.

Mom's Chicken Soup

Sometimes called Jewish penicillin, chicken soup has been used to soothe flu and colds since the twelfth century.

1 chicken (3 to 4 pounds, or 1.4 to 1.8 kg), fully washed

2 quarts (2 L) water

1 large onion, peeled and quartered

6 carrots, grated, divided

4 garlic cloves, peeled, minced, divided

1 can (28 ounces, or 80 g) crushed tomatoes

2 celery stalks, sliced thinly

1 cup (90 g) uncooked bow-tie pasta

Freshly ground black pepper

2 tablespoons (8 g) fresh dill

PREPARATION AND USE:

Place the chicken in a large pot and cover it with the water.
Add the onion, three of the chopped carrots, and two of the minced garlic cloves. Bring the water to a boil, then turn down the heat, cover the pot, and simmer for about an hour. When the chicken is cooked through, remove it to let cool. Pour the broth through a strainer and throw away (or compost) the vegetables. Return the broth to the original pot. Skin the chicken, tear it apart, and add the pieces to the pot. Add the tomatoes, celery, and the three remaining chopped carrots. Stir in the pasta, ground pepper, and dill. Cook until the pasta is tender enough to eat. Add the remaining two minced garlic cloves. Serve warm.

YIELD: 8 servings

? How it works: For eight hundred years, chicken soup has headed the list of flu relievers. Recent scientific evidence shows mild support for the notion that chicken soup reduces congestion and other cold symptoms. Drinking warm liquids will keep you hydrated and help ease a sore throat; the steam helps to clear nasal passages. Add garlic at the end of the cooking time to take advantage of its immune-enhancing and flu-fighting ingredients, which heat destroys. Dill relaxes smooth muscle—the kind that encircles the lower airways, which may help ease chest tightness.

Fact or Myth?

STARVE A FEVER; FEED A COLD.

Myth. If you want to get better, you have to eat right. Listen to your body and eat when you feel like it. Simple food helps your body heal, so eat foods that you can digest, such as broths, rice, and soft proteins. And drink plenty of fluids to replace those you've lost through fever, coughing, and congestion.

Elderberry Syrup

Most herb stores and online bulk herb retailers carry European black elderberries (Sambucus nigra). American elderberry (S. canadensis), which is similar, grows in some regions of the United States. Verify the species of local varieties before consuming. Use only ripe, black elderberries, never red elderberries, which are poisonous.

3 cups (710 ml) water

1 cup (120 g) dried elderberries

2 tablespoons (28 g) cinnamon chips, from
a crushed cinnamon stick

1 tablespoon (8 g) fresh, grated ginger, or
2 teaspoons (4 g) dried

¾ cup (240 g) honey

2 teaspoons (10 ml) brandy

PREPARATION AND USE:

Bring the water to a boil in a quart-size (946 ml) saucepan. Add the elderberries, cinnamon chips, and ginger. Lower the heat and simmer, uncovered, for 40 minutes. The water level should reduce by almost half, but you should still have enough water to adequately cover the herbs. Drape a piece of cheesecloth over a large strainer and balance it atop a glass measuring cup or a bowl. Strain the herbs. Fold the cheesecloth around the herbs and wring out the remaining liquid. If you have more than 1½ cups (355 ml) of liquid, return it to the pot and simmer until it reduces to 1½ cups (355 ml). Add the honey. (To make a syrup, the ratio of strong tea to honey should be 2:1.) Stir to blend. If the liquid is warm, the honey should dissolve easily. If not, return to heat until it does. Add a splash (about 2 teaspoons [10 ml]) of brandy to preserve. Refrigerate. The mixture is good for three months. At the first sign of influenza (or after a recent exposure), take 1 tablespoon (15 ml) four times a day. Give children half that dose. This remedy is not appropriate for infants.

YIELD: Multiple servings

❓ **How it works:** European black elderberries (*Sambucus nigra*) have immune-enhancing and antiviral activity against influenza and other respiratory viruses. Three small studies have demonstrated that special elderberry extracts reduced symptom severity and duration in people with influenza. The first two studies used a proprietary extract sold as Sambucol. The dose was 4 tablespoons (60 ml) a day for adults, and 2 tablespoons (30 ml) a day for children. Cinnamon and ginger are warming, pleasant tasting, immune-enhancing, and antioxidant. Ginger inhibits some respiratory viruses, though it may not fight influenza viruses. It also counters inflammation, fever, pain, and cough—all of which can accompany the flu.

❗ **Warning:** The seeds of unripe elderberries contain substances called cyanogenic glycosides, which, if ingested can be toxic. Red elderberries are poisonous.

Recipe Variation: You can also make this syrup without the brandy and use as a delicious topping to yogurt, oatmeal, and pancakes.

Musculoskeletal Pain, Arthritis, Joint Swelling

— and —

Sprains

Pain is a useful sensory perception. Without it, you might continue walking after a tack punctured your foot. Or, you might arise from a skiing accident and continue downhill with a ruptured ligament. Pain alerts you to injury and forces you to lie low until you recover.

Chronic pain is another story. If you have arthritis (joint degeneration), you're well aware of the problem. Not using the joint can actually further the deterioration. Yet the ache holds you back. In this case, a visual cue—perhaps a change in the color of your fingernails—seems kinder and equally helpful. When it's time to rest, your fingernails would glow a fire engine red.

A number of maladies can cause discomfort in muscles and joints. We're going to focus on two things: traumatic injuries and osteoarthritis. Mechanical trauma can hurt all elements of the musculoskeletal system: muscles, the tendons that attach muscle to bone, the ligaments that hold the joints together, the joints, and the bones.

To a lesser extent, overuse can injure the musculoskeletal system. Many people who use a computer keyboard have experienced tendinitis (tendon inflammation). "Weekend warriors"—relatively inactive people who decide to jog 10 miles (16 kilometers) or play three sets of tennis on Saturday—also know the signs and symptoms.

After a rigorous workout, it's not uncommon to experience muscle soreness the next day. Unless the pain is severe, consider this discomfort a sign of weakness leaving your body. What's happened is that high-intensity workouts cause microscopic tears in muscle fibers. The muscle then rebuilds and gains bulk. The repair process makes it stronger. Strains and sprains are ailments that occur at any age. Strains occur when a muscle or the tendon that attaches it to the bone becomes pulled or twisted. They can occur suddenly (such as from shoveling snow) or over a longer period from overuse.

RECIPES TO PREVENT AND MANAGE MUSCLE AND JOINT PAIN

Ice It

I learned this method from a physical therapist when I had "tennis elbow." It really helped. ~ LBW

Water
Small paper cups

PREPARATION AND USE:

Pour water into 6 small paper cups and set them on a shelf in the freezer. Once the water has frozen, remove a cup. Starting at the top of the cup, peel away a strip of paper wide enough to expose the ice. The remaining paper protects your fingers from the cold. Briskly massage the inflamed area with the ice for 3 to 5 minutes. (Do not hold the ice stationary on the same spot; doing so can eventually freeze tissue, damaging it.) If it's a tendon, passing the ice across the fiber (perpendicular to its length) enhances mobility.

YIELD: 6 servings

❓ **How it works:** The cold reduces inflammation.

LIFESTYLE TIP

A number of gadgets can reduce the stress on your joints. Rubber grips on gardening tools, pens, and kitchen appliances increase comfort. Try placing a rubber band around twist-off tops for jars, bottles, and tubes (e.g., toothpaste) to make it easier to open them. Long-handled grippers can help you grab objects.

Avo-Kale Arthritis Arrester

1½ cups (100 g) washed, chopped kale, divided

⅛ teaspoon salt

Juice of 1 lime

1 avocado, pitted, peeled, and cut into chunks

1 tomato, chopped and seeded

1 carrot, grated

¼ cup (25 g) pitted and chopped green olives

1 garlic clove, minced

¼ cup (36 g) cashews

2 tablespoons (8 g) chopped fresh flat-leaf parsley or (2 g) cilantro leaves

Freshly ground black pepper

PREPARATION AND USE:

In a large bowl, sprinkle 1 cup (67 g) of the kale with the salt and massage the kale leaves for a minute or so until they begin to wilt. Transfer the kale to a colander to rinse off the salt and then return the kale to the bowl. Drizzle in the lime juice and massage again so that the kale is covered with the juice. Add the avocado, gently tossing it with the kale while maintaining the avocado's chunkiness. Mix in the remaining kale, along with the tomato, carrot, olives, garlic, and cashews. Sprinkle in the parsley, add the pepper, and toss gently. Divide between two plates and serve.

YIELD: 2 servings

❓ How it works: Brightly colored fruits and vegetables, such as kale, avocado, tomato, carrot, and green olives, indicate the presence of antioxidant and anti-inflammatory flavonoids and carotenoids. The oil in avocados—called the "unsaponifiable fractions"—has been found to improve pain and disability of osteoarthritis.

Turmeric-Ginger Inflammation Fighter

I rely on these antioxidant, anti-inflammatory, pain-relieving spices to counter the inevitable aches and pains of a an active lifestyle and—let's face it—an aging body. ~ LBW

1 tablespoon (6 g) minced fresh ginger,
or 1½ teaspoons (3 g) dried

1 teaspoon (2 g) ground turmeric

½ teaspoon ground cumin

$1/8$ teaspoon freshly ground black pepper

¼ teaspoon cayenne pepper

1 cup (235 ml) vegetable or chicken stock

1 tablespoon (15 ml) sesame oil

½ cup (80 g) chopped onion

2 cups (142 g) broccoli florets

1 cup (130 g) thinly sliced carrot

1 seeded and diced red bell pepper

1 cup (70 g) sliced shiitake mushrooms

1 cup (230 g) cubed tofu

2 cups (134 g) washed and torn kale, packed

2 garlic cloves, minced

2 tablespoons (2 g) fresh cilantro leaves, for garnish

4 cups (780 g) cooked brown rice (optional)

PREPARATION AND USE:

In a small bowl, mix the ginger, turmeric, cumin, black and cayenne pepper, and stock. Heat the sesame oil in a skillet or wok over medium heat. Sauté the onion for 3 to 5 minutes until soft. Add the herb-laced stock and stir for 3 minutes. Add the broccoli, carrot, bell pepper, mushrooms, and tofu. Cover the pan. Simmer the vegetables for 3 to 5 minutes until the broccoli turns a brilliant green. Add the kale and garlic. Cook over low heat for 1 to 2 more minutes. Garnish with cilantro leaves. Serve alone or over brown rice.

YIELD: Serves 4

❓ **How it works:** Brightly colored vegetables contain antioxidant and anti-inflammatory flavonoids and carotenoids. Turmeric, the spice that makes curry yellow, contains the potent anti-inflammatory chemical curcumin. Studies show specially prepared curcumin supplements have helped ease arthritis pain. Ginger, which belongs to the same plant family as turmeric, decreases pain and inflammation. In one study, 250 milligrams four times a day of a ginger extract diminished pain from knee osteoarthritis, but only after three months of continuous use.

LIFESTYLE TIP

Consider magnets. For people with osteoarthritis in the hip or knee, a few studies have shown that wearing magnets helped relieve joint pain more effectively than a placebo. However, it's hard to know whether the magnetic bracelets, necklaces, and pads on the retail market are as strong as those used in studies. There is interest in magnet therapy because the body has natural electromagnetic fields that researchers think may react positively to magnets. For instance, muscle contractions induced by signals from the nervous system are linked to magnetic activity. There is not yet enough information on exactly how magnets work to relieve pain, but researchers note that such products seem to do no harm.

Muscle-Boosting Beet & Tart Cherry Tonic

1 cup (155 g) fresh tart cherries, stemmed,
pitted, and halved, or (245 g) frozen or canned cherries
2 apples, peeled, cored, and cut into chunks
¼ cup (60 ml) beet juice, or 1 small beet peeled and chopped
3 to 4 ice cubes

PREPARATION AND USE:
Put the cherries and apples into a blender. Add the beet juice or chopped
beet and ice. Blend. Drink for a muscle tune-up.

YIELD: 2 small servings or 1 large serving

❓ **How it works:** Cherries contain a number of antioxidant and anti-inflammatory flavonoids. Studies have shown that tart cherry juice prevents weakness and pain that might otherwise follow a bout of intense exercise. Another trial found that consuming cherry juice (relative to a placebo juice) five days before a marathon and continuing for the day of the event and two days afterward reduced muscle inflammation and promoted recovery.

Eating cherries also helps. Two studies found that eating forty-five cherries a day decreased blood levels of the body's inflammatory chemicals. Another showed that people with gout who ate cherries had fewer attacks of painful arthritis. Researchers have shown that drinking beet juice may improve athlete performance by enhancing the efficiency of skeletal muscles' use of oxygen. As a side benefit, blood pressure was also reduced.

Note: Beet juice is available at natural food stores or online. As a quick alternative, add 1 cup (235 ml) of pomegranate juice to 1 cup (245 g) of canned tart cherries and blend. Yum!

Muscle Approach by Poach

2 ounces (946 ml) extra-virgin olive oil, with or without flavoring

garlic cloves, crushed

teaspoon (2 g) freshly ground black pepper

teaspoon (3 g) paprika

tablespoons (8 g) fresh chopped fresh dill

bay leaves

salmon steaks (4 ounces, or 115 g)

PREPARATION AND USE:

Preheat the oven to 300°F (150°C, or gas mark 2). Fill a baking pan halfway with water and place on the lower rack of the oven (this will keep the fish moist). Pour the oil into a cast-iron skillet on the stove. Heat the oil over low heat, stirring in the garlic, pepper, paprika, dill, and bay leaves until the oil simmers. Add the salmon and spoon the herbed oil over the steaks, ensuring that they are fully covered by the oil. Allow the oil to return to a simmer. Remove the pan from the stove and place in the oven on the middle rack, above the pan of water. Bake for about 15 minutes. The salmon is ready when it flakes with a fork. Do not overcook.

YIELD: 4 servings

❓ How it works: Extra-virgin olive oil and cold-water fish, both part of the Mediterranean diet, contain fats with anti-inflammatory effects. The Mediterranean diet reduces inflammation and may be helpful in people with rheumatoid arthritis. Fish oil supplements also reduce morning stiffness associated with rheumatoid arthritis.

Cooling Muscle Balm

2 tablespoons (30 g) Aloe vera gel

8 to 10 drops peppermint essential oil

PREPARATION AND USE:

Blend the aloe and oil in a small, clean bowl. Massage the mixture into sore muscles. Wash your hands afterward and avoid getting it in your eyes.

YIELD: 1 application

❓ How it works: Peppermint contains menthol, which, when applied topically, causes a cooling sensation and is thought to inhibit pain receptors.

Warning: Some people are sensitive to peppermint essential oil. If you develop skin irritation, discontinue use.

Note: Apply to a small area first to adjust the amount of the peppermint to your liking.

LIFESTYLE TIP

Stretch three times a week. Slowly move your joints through their complete range of motion. Doing so helps to maintain flexibility and reduces the risk of injury.

Nausea
— and —
Vomiting

Nausea and vomiting are common and stem from multiple causes. Like diarrhea, vomiting represents a nonspecific defense to rid the body of noxious substances. Culprits include alcohol intoxication, injudicious eating, food allergies and intolerances, food poisoning, microbes that infect the gastrointestinal tract, and chemotherapy. Sometimes there isn't anything nasty to expel. Take, for example, motion sickness and morning sickness in pregnancy. Migraine headaches can produce nausea, and the headache may subside after a bout of vomiting.

Regardless of the cause, the symptoms are certainly unpleasant. Here are some tips for managing the situation:

- Rest your stomach. Let your stomach empty itself before you put anything in. A good rule of thumb is to wait 8 hours before attempting solid foods.

- After 1 to 2 hours, begin drinking small amounts of clear fluids. Stretching the stomach may cause reflex vomiting, so even if you're thirsty, start with sips. Children may need to be given fluids by the spoonful. (If your child is under twelve months of age, call your pediatrician for advice.)

- If those first fluids do cause vomiting, wait another hour or two before trying again.

- Stay hydrated. That can be difficult when you can only drink tiny amounts—but keep at it. Sip frequently. Dehydration causes nausea, which may lead to vomiting, which increases your fluid losses. Dehydration also increases body temperature, which further increases fluid losses. And it can give you a headache.

- Don't rely on plain water as your main rehydration fluid. You've lost electrolytes and other bodily chemicals.

- Steer clear of dairy products for at least twenty-four hours.

- After 8 hours of clear liquids (and no more vomiting), try bland foods such as pasta, rice, saltine crackers, bananas, applesauce, and cooked carrots.

Rice Water

3 cups (710 ml) water

$^1/8$ teaspoon (0.75 g) salt

¼ cup (49 g) uncooked white rice

1 tablespoon (9 g) raisins

1 teaspoon (3 g) grated fresh ginger

Honey, to taste

PREPARATION AND USE:

In a medium-size saucepan, combine water, salt, and rice. Bring to a boil. Lower the heat. Stir in the raisins and ginger, and then cover. Cook over low heat for an hour. Pour through a strainer into a mug. Set aside the rice and raisins for when you're keeping down clear liquids. Allow the rice water to cool. Add honey or salt as desired, and sip.

YIELD: 1 serving

❓ **How it works:** This traditional Asian remedy can help replace the water, sugars, and salts your body has lost. Ginger is the best-researched antinausea agent.

Note: For a nutritious soup, add ½ cup (120 ml) vegetable or chicken stock to the rice water and ½ cup (93 g) of the strained rice.

Congee

This rice porridge is traditionally used in Asian countries.

1½ quarts (1.4 L) water

1 cup (185 g) uncooked long-grain white rice

1 teaspoon (6 g) salt

PREPARATION AND USE:

In a large pot, mix the water and rice. Bring the mixture to a boil. Cover, tilting the lid to release steam. Lower the heat to its lowest setting. Cook for 4 hours, stirring occasionally, until the rice is very soft and creamy. Stir in the salt.

YIELD: Various, depending on size. Eat a little at a time, as the stomach allows.

❓ **How it works:** This soft rice is easy to digest and returns water and salt to the depleted system.

Soup-er Broth

This soup is nourishing, tasty, and easy to digest.

2 cups (475 ml) water

2 chicken bouillon cubes

2 teaspoons (4 g) minced fresh ginger

Pinch of ground cinnamon

PREPARATION AND USE:

In a small saucepan, boil the water with the bouillon cubes, stirring until dissolved. Add the ginger and cook over low heat for 30 minutes. Strain out the ginger. Serve with a pinch of cinnamon.

YIELD: 2 servings

? **How it works:** Bouillon broth returns salt and other nutrients to the depleted system. Ginger and cinnamon can also help settle the stomach.

Note: For a nutritious soup, add ½ cup (120 ml) vegetable or chicken stock to the rice water and ½ cup (93 g) of the strained rice.

Zingy Minty Nausea Fighter

I like this tea because the ginger and mint work together to fight nausea.
~ LBW

2 cups (475 ml) water

2 teaspoons (1 g) dried peppermint or spearmint leaves,
   or 1 tablespoon (6 g) fresh

1 teaspoon (3 g) grated fresh ginger, or

½ teaspoon dried

1 teaspoon (7 g) honey

PREPARATION AND USE:

In a saucepan, bring the water to a boil. Add the peppermint and ginger.
Turn off the heat, cover, and steep for 15 minutes. Strain out the herbs.
Stir in the honey. Sip frequently.

YIELD: Various, depending on size. Eat a little at a time, as the stomach allows.

❓ **How it works:** The prime antinausea agent ginger combines with
mint, which also reduces nausea and generally helps settle the stomach.

❗ **Warning:** Do not give honey to children under twelve months of age.
Use molasses, pure maple syrup, or raw sugar instead.

Note: Alternatively, use tea bags instead of fresh leaves. Also, you can
double the recipe and set aside to sip continuously throughout the day.

Stomach-Settling Tea

This tea can be particularly comforting if you're feeling chilled.

2 cups (475 ml) water

1 teaspoon (2 g) dried ginger, or 2 teaspoons (5 g) grated fresh

¾ teaspoon aniseeds

¼ teaspoon ground cardamom

Honey

PREPARATION AND USE:

In a small saucepan, bring water to a boil. Turn heat to low. Add spices and stir. Simmer for 5 minutes. Cover and steep for 20 minutes. Strain. Add honey, if desired. Sip slowly.

YIELD: 2 servings

❓ **How it works:** Ginger combats nausea. Anise and cardamom reduce intestinal spasm if your nausea is accompanied by diarrhea.

WHEN SIMPLE DOESN'T WORK

Severe nausea and vomiting, such as that associated with cancer chemotherapy, can require prescription medications. Regardless of the cause, severe, repeated vomiting may require intravenous fluids to correct dehydration.

Rehydrate and Restore

This recipe is adapted from the Rehydration Project, a global organization that fights dehydration through simple, accessible treatments. It predicts that this and other home-based solutions can help save the lives of some 2 million children each year.

1 level teaspoon (6 g) salt

8 level teaspoons (22 g) sugar

5 cups (1.2 L) clean water (If unsure, boil and then cool.)

½ cup (120 ml) orange juice, or ¼ cup (56 g) mashed banana

PREPARATION AND USE:

Stir the salt and sugar into the water until fully dissolved. Whisk in the orange juice or banana until fully blended. Take slowly, by the teaspoonful (5 ml), ingesting as much as possible after a vomiting or diarrheal episode. If another episode takes place, wait 10 minutes and then begin taking the solution again.

YIELD: Multiple applications

❓ **How it works:** Starch, sugar, sodium, and potassium return vital nutrients to the body after depletion by vomiting, diarrhea, or other loss of fluids. They also help the body retain essential fluids and salts when another episode takes place.

Note: Store in a cool place. This solution is good for about twenty-four hours. After that time, prepare a fresh one. Take additional liquids to help restore hydration.

Sore Throat

You know that scratchy feeling that gets worse when you try to swallow. Sometimes a raw throat is the first sign of the common cold or other respiratory infection. Other agents can irritate the throat, too: hot liquids, chemicals, smoke, allergies, postnasal drip from sinusitis, and even sleeping with your mouth open at night.

Viruses—particularly those associated with the common cold—are far and away the most common infectious cause. Normally, other respiratory symptoms, such as runny nose and sneezing, accompany the throat pain. Viral sore throat should resolve on its own within a few days.

Another viral illness that starts with a sore throat is mononucleosis, a condition that typically strikes teens and young adults. In addition to severe sore throat, signs and symptoms include extreme fatigue, malaise, decreased appetite, chills, fever, body aches, swollen lymph nodes in the neck, enlarged spleen, and sensitivity to light. The Epstein-Barr virus is the cause. It spreads from close contact with infected saliva or respiratory mucus—hence the illness's nickname "the kissing disease."

Bacteria can also infect the throat, particularly *Streptococcus pyogenes*, the cause of strep throat. The onset of sore throat is sudden, with pain on swallowing, tender and swollen lymph nodes in the neck, fever, headache, and possibly nausea and vomiting (especially in children). Unless you have the bad luck of also having a cold, a runny nose, sneezing, and cough are absent. Doctors treat strep throat with antibiotics.

Sore Throat Tea

Down this tangy throat soother while the honey is still warm.

1 cup (235 ml) water
1 tablespoon (2 g) fresh thyme leaves
1 tablespoon (4 g) fresh oregano leaves
1 tablespoon (3 g) fresh sage leaves

PREPARATION AND USE:
Boil the water in the bottom of a double boiler. Place the other ingredients in the top of the double boiler. Gently heat the honey mixture for 30 to 60 minutes. Strain through a tea strainer. (You'll get about ¼ cup [60 ml] or less.) Drink right away while still warm.

YIELD: About ¼ cup (60 ml), just enough to coat the throat

? **How it works:** Honey is antibacterial, soothing, and moistening. The three herbs are antimicrobial. With heat, you've infused the honey with the herb's healing chemicals.

LIFESTYLE TIP

Cranberry juice is a great gargle and an even better drink. It contains salicylic acid (the backbone chemical of aspirin), which eases inflammation and pain in the throat.

Homemade Neck Cozy

cups (about 540 g) rice, dried lentils, millet, barley, or other microwave-safe grain

o drops lavender, peppermint, eucalyptus, or other essential oil

REPARATION AND USE:

'our the grain into a bowl, sprinkle the essential oil over it, and mix. 'our the scented grain into a clean tube sock. Leave enough room to knot he open end of the sock. (You can also sew it closed.) Microwave on high or 60 to 90 seconds.

Check the temperature: It should feel pleasantly warm to the touch but not calding hot. Wrap the sock around your neck. Ideally, you should do this fter the neck massage described in the previous recipe. Sip warm tea nd relax.

'IELD: 1 application

❷ **How it works:** Heat increases local circulation, which increases the delivery of immune cells and the removal of wastes. It also feels good. The essential oils are antimicrobial, smell nice, and help clear a stuffy nose that accompanies your sore throat.

Apple-Cinnamon Toddy

While you reap the benefits of the apple and spices, the warm liquid helps soothe an irritated throat and loosen congestion.

1 quart (946 ml) apple juice or cider
1 quart (946 ml) water (to dilute the sugar in the juice)
1 cinnamon stick
3 or 4 whole cloves
½ teaspoon ground ginger
Fresh lemon juice

PREPARATION AND USE:

Pour the juice and water into a large pan. Add the spices. Heat until just beginning to boil. Turn the heat to low, stirring occasionally. Simmer for 30 minutes. Strain out the cinnamon stick and cloves. Enjoy each cup with a squirt of lemon juice.

YIELD: 4 servings

❓ **How it works:** You're delivering warmth and antimicrobial plant chemicals to your throat, which both soothe and heal it. Ginger is especially warming, antiviral, anti-inflammatory, and pain relieving.

Sage and Thyme Gargle

1 cup (235 ml) water
1 tablespoon (3 g) dried thyme
2 teaspoons (2 g) dried sage
1 teaspoon (6 g) salt

PREPARATION AND USE:

Bring the water to a boil in a small pan. Stir in the thyme and sage. Cover and steep for 20 minutes. Strain. Reheat, if necessary. (You want the water as hot as you can stand it without burning.) Add the salt and stir. Gargle and spit out. Continue until you finish the cup. Repeat four to five times a day, making a hot, fresh batch each time.

YIELD: 1 application

❓ **How it works:** Sage and thyme are antioxidant and antimicrobial.